SPECIAL TOPICS IN RESUSCITATION

Edited by **Theodoros K. Aslanidis**

Special Topics in Resuscitation
http://dx.doi.org/10.5772/intechopen.74766
Edited by Theodoros K. Aslanidis

Contributors

Georg Schmolzer, Francesca Viaroli, Digna M González-Otero, Sofía Ruiz De Gauna, Jose Julio Gutiérrez, Purificación Saiz, Jesus M Ruiz, Alain Frederic Kalmar, Nicky Van Der Vekens, Jan Heerman, Henk Vanoverschelde, Anton Kasatkin, Aleksandr Urakov, Anna Nigmatullina, Theodoros Aslanidis

First published in London, United Kingdom, 2018 by IntechOpen
IntechOpen is the global imprint of INTECHOPEN LIMITED, registered in England and Wales, registration number: 11086078, The Shard, 25th floor, 32 London Bridge Street
London, SE19SG – United Kingdom
Printed in Croatia

British Library Cataloguing-in-Publication Data
A catalogue record for this book is available from the British Library

Additional hard copies can be obtained from orders@intechopen.com

Special Topics in Resuscitation, Edited by Theodoros K. Aslanidis
p. cm.
Print ISBN 978-1-78984-251-7
Online ISBN 978-1-78984-252-4

For EU product safety concerns:
IN TECH d.o.o., Prolaz Marije Krucifikse Kozulić 3, 51000 Rijeka, Croatia,
info@intechopen.com or visit our website at intechopen.com.

Meet the editor

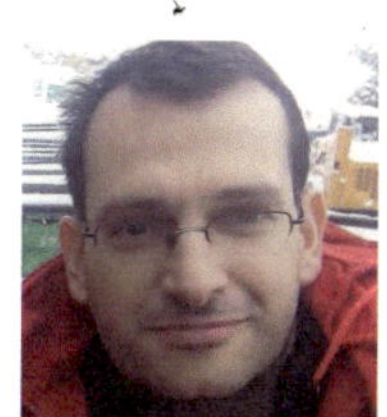

Dr. Theodoros K. Aslanidis received his Doctor of Medicine degree from the Plovdiv Medical University, Bulgaria and his PhD degree from the Aristotle University of Thessaloniki, Greece. After serving in the Hellenic Army Force as a medical doctor, he worked as a rural physician at the Outhealth Centre, Iraklia and Serres General Hospital, Greece. He completed his residency in Anaesthesiology from the "Hippokratio" General Hospital of Thessaloniki, followed by fellowship training in Critical Care at the AHEPA University Hospital, and a postgraduate program in Prehospital Emergency Medicine. He served as an EMS Physician and Emergency Communication Centre Medic at Hellenic National Centre for Emergency Care before moving to his current post as a consultant-researcher at the Intensive Care Unit of St. Paul General Hospital of Thessaloniki, Greece. His research interests are medical writing, data analysis, critical emergency medicine, neurosonology, and electrodermal activity.

Contents

Preface

Over 50 years have passed since the proposed "close chest cardiac massage" by Kouwenhoven and the "race against the D(eath)-time," and the challenge for better outcomes remains. On one hand, we have moved to a more holistic approach—from cardiac massage to cardiopulmonary resuscitation (CPR) to advance life support (ALS), while research on a more personalized approach is growing.

Today, assisted-device CPR, alternative CPR position, e.g. prone-CPR, patient-centric blood pressure targeted CPR, flow-enhanced CPR, neuroprotection during resuscitation, new training methods in resource-limited health systems, implementation of phone-assister CPR, and implantation of venoarterial extracorporeal membrane oxygenation (VA-ECMO), the so-called E-CPR, are only some of the issues currently being researched.

Within this frame, this book, published by IntechOpen, comes as a natural sequel after the previous publications on the subject. Divided into two sections, it focuses on specific resuscitation topics from the role of the physician in prehospital care to possible future applications, such as the use of transthoracic impedance in the field.

The authors offer the reader not only a "vigorous" review of the current literature but also a research path for further advancement. A path proves that resuscitation is anything but an exhausted subject for both the clinician and the researcher.

Theodoros K. Aslanidis MD, PhD
Anesthesiology-Intensive Care
Pre hospital Emergency Medicine
Intensive Care Unit
St. Paul General Hospital
Thessaloniki, Greece

Section 1

Introduction

Chapter 1

Introductory Chapter: The Role of Emergency Medical Service Physician

Theodoros Aslanidis

Additional information is available at the end of the chapter

http://dx.doi.org/10.5772/intechopen.80916

1. Introduction: emergency medical services as medical subspecialty

Almost 45 years since the inception of first modern emergency medical services (EMS) in the United States with the Highway Safety Act of 1966 and the EMS Services Development Act of 1973 [1, 2], the American Board of Medical Specialties (ABMS) voted in 2011 to create a new physician subspecialty called "emergency medical services" [3]. The American Board of Emergency Medicine was named the parent board for this subspecialty and held its first board certification exam in 2013.

The first suggestions about an EMS subspecialty head back to late 1990s by the creation of an ABEM task force and later, in 2001, by National Association of Emergency Medical Society Physicians (NAEMSP's EMS Physician) Certification Task Force. Yet, it took another ten years and the continuous tremendous advance in prehospital care in the last decades that finally led to the new emergency medicine subspecialty [4].

Today, the list of the existing subspecialties of emergency medicine [5] is:

- anesthesiology critical care medicine,
- emergency medical services,
- hospice and palliative medicine,
- internal medicine-critical care medicine,
- medical toxicology,
- pain medicine,
- pediatric emergency medicine,

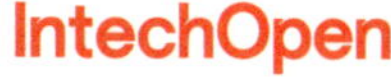

- sports medicine, and
- undersea and hyperbaric medicine;

thus covering almost all kinds of emergency medical care.

However, outside US, emergency medical systems are considered a relative new addition to the Healthcare systems [2]. Even now (2018), the state of EMS still varies drastically from developed to developing countries [6].

Within the aforementioned frame, the present article aims at describing the possible roles of the EMS physician.

2. The role of EMS physician

2.1. On scene

EMS personnel are recognized as the extension of the physician in the field, a "delegated practitioner." Even though the current level of training in other EMS personnel (EMTs, Paramedics) is continuously raising, active involvement of the physicians in prehospital emergency care of patients is still needed.

There are several studies about out-of-hospital cardiac arrest (OHCA), synthesized in a recent meta-analysis [7], that suggests that EMS-physician-guided CPR in OHCA is associated with improved survival outcomes. Yet, due to the fact that the meta-analysis is based solely on observational studies, some authors doubt its results [8]. The same dispute is ongoing when it comes to single country studies about the same subject [9]. On the contrary, in cases of traumatic OHCA and in cases of severe injured patients, the presence of an EMS physician on the field is related with increased survival [10–12].

2.2. Beyond direct patient care

The high level of EMS personnel allows the system to work, most of the time, independently on the scene. Yet, the role of EMS physician extent beyond direct patient care; as he can serve as a coordinator or team leader, as an EMS educator, as the legal component of the system, as the patient advocate, or as the link between EMS and the hospital health care [13].

Thus, EMS physician can serve as the ideal Medical Director that can provide management, supervision, and guidance in an effort to assure quality of care [14]. The recent American College of Emergency Physicians (ACEP) policy statement gives the main principles of the role [15].

2.3. The challenge for the best EMS physicians' utilization

Though recognition of EMS subspecialty seems to create a new dynamic in prehospital emergency medicine, the optimum way of utilization of EMS physicians remains a question.

Even in the US, EMS agencies have significant practice variability with regard to quality improvement resources, medical direction, and specific clinical quality measures [16]. At the same time, there is a lack of share in understanding of which quality indicators to be used by physician-staffed EMS [17]. The heterogeneity of EMS systems in terms of organization (Anglo-American concept or European), equipment availability, staffing (EMTs, paramedics, EMS physicians, anesthesiologists, etc.), and level of training, on the one hand, and the national or regional determinants of prehospital healthcare system (geographical, socioeconomic factors, etc.), on the other hand, make it even harder to find the answer.

The formation of a self-regulatory quality improvement system (SQIS) with flexible model of best human recourse utilization, adapted to the data feedback from the local or regional characteristics of EMS utilization, may be the most prudent way for resolving the problem.

Conflict of interests

The author has no conflict of interest.

Author details

Theodoros Aslanidis

Address all correspondence to: thaslan@hotmail.com

Intensive Care Unit, St. Paul General Hospital of Thessaloniki, Thessaloniki, Greece

References

[1] Emergency Medical Services Systems Development Act of 1973. Hearings. 93rd Congress, 1st Session, on §504.and §654. Washington, DC: United States Congress, Senate, Committee on Labor and Public Welfare, Subcommittee on Health; 1973. pp. 691-694

[2] Shah MN. The formation of the emergency medical services system. American Journal of Public Health. 2006;**96**(3):414-423. DOI: 10.2105/AJPH.2004.048793

[3] American Board of Medical Specialties. Emergency Medical Services: Eligibility Vriteria for Certification. 2011. Available from: http://www.naemsp.org/Documents/EMSEligCriteriaFINALApril2011.pdf [Accessed: 9-7-2018]

[4] Escott M. EMS Subspecialty creates an opportunity to change the role of the paramedic. JEMS: A Journal of Emergency Medical Services. 2015;**40**(1). https://www.jems.com/articles/print/volume-40/issue-1/departments-columns/field-physicians/ems-subspecialty-creates-opportunity-cha.html [Accessed: 10-7-2018]

[5] American Board of Medical Specialties. Specialty and Subspecialty Certificates. 2011. Available from: https://www.abms.org/member-boards/specialty-subspecialty-certificates [Accessed: 10-7-2018]

[6] Aslanidis T. EMS Health Staff Problems: Facts and Solution: Asian Hospital Healthcare & Management. 2018. Available from: https://www.asianhhm.com/articles/ems-staff-health-problems [Accessed: 08-07-2018]

[7] Bottiger BW, Berhhard M, Knapp J, Nagele P. Influence of EMS-physician presence on survival after out-of-hospital cardiopulmonary resuscitation: Systematic review and meta-analysis. Critical Care. 2016;**20**:4. DOI: 10.1186/s13054-015-1156-6

[8] Von Vopelious-Feld J, Benger J. Response to: Influence of EMS-physician presence on survival after out-of-hospital cardiopulmonary resuscitation. Critical Care. 2016;**20**:324. DOI: 10.1186/s13054-016-1495-y

[9] Fouche P, Jennings PA. Physician presence at out-of-hospital cardiac arrest is not necessarily the cause of improved survival. Scandinavian Journal of Trauma, Resuscitation and Emergency Medicine. 2016;**24**(1):88. DOI: 10.1186/s13049-016-282-8

[10] Fjaeldstad A, Kirk MH, Knudsen L, Bjerring J, Christensen EF. Physician-staffed emergency helicopter reduces transportation time from alarm call to highly specialized centre. Danish Medical Journal. 2013;**60**(7):A4666

[11] Den Hartog D, Romeo J, Ringburg AN, Verhofstad MH, Van Lieshout EM. Survival benefit of physician-staffed helicopter emergency medical services (HEMS) assistance for severely injured patients. Injury. 2015;**46**(7):1281-1286. DOI: 10.1016/j.injury.2015.04.013

[12] Fukuda T, Ohashi-Fukuda N, Kondo Y, Hayashida K, Kukita I. Association of prehospital advanced life support by physician with survival after out-of-hospital cardiac arrest with blunt trauma following traffic collisions: Japanese registry-based study. JAMA Surgery. 2018;**153**(6):e180674. DOI: 10.1001/jamasurg.2018.0674

[13] American College of Emergency Physicians (ACEP); National Association Of EMS Physicians (NAEMSP); National Association Of State EMS Officials (NASEMSO). Role of the state EMS medical director. Prehospital Emergency Care 2010;**14**(3):402. DOI: 10.3109/10903121003770688

[14] Munjal KG. The Role of the medical director: A more collaborative, multidisciplinary oversight is called for in the future. EMS World. 2016;Suppl:10-11

[15] American College of Emergency Physicians. The Role of the Physician Medical Director in Emergency Medical Services Leadership: Policy Statement. 2017. Available from: https://www.acep.org/globalassets/new-pdfs/policy-statements/the.role.of.the.physician.medical.director.in.ems.leadership.pdf [Accessed: 06-08-2018]

[16] Redenier M, Olivieri P, Loo GT, Muniai K, Hilton MT, Potkin KT, et al. National assessment of quality programs in emergency medical services. Prehospital Emergency Care. 2018;**22**(3):370-378. DOI: 10.1080/10903127.2017.1800094

[17] Haugland H, Uleberg O, Klepstad P, Kruger A, Rehn M. Quality measurement in physician-staffed emergency medical services: A systematic literature review. International Journal for Quality in Health Care. 2018;**30**(4). DOI: 10.1093/intqhc/mzy106

Section 2

Special Topics

Chapter 2

Managing the Prevention of In-Hospital Resuscitation by Early Detection and Treatment of High-Risk Patients

Alain Kalmar, Nicky Van Der Vekens,
Henk Vanoverschelde, Diederik Van Sassenbroeck,
Jan Heerman and Tom Verbeke

Additional information is available at the end of the chapter

http://dx.doi.org/10.5772/intechopen.79651

Abstract

In hospitalized patients, cardiorespiratory collapse mostly occurs after a distinct period of deterioration. This deterioration can be discovered by a systematic quantification of a set of clinical parameters. The combination of such a detection system—to identify patients at risk in an early stage —and a rapid response team—which can intervene immediately—can be implemented to prevent life-threatening situations and reduce the incidence of in-hospital cardiac arrests outside the intensive care setting. The effectiveness of both of these systems is influenced by the used trigger criteria, the number of rapid response team (RRT) activations, the in- or exclusion of patients with a DNR code >3, proactive rounding, the team composition, and its response time. Each of those elements should be optimized for maximal efficacy, and both systems need to work in tandem with little delay between patient deterioration, accurate detection, and swift intervention. Dependable diagnostics and scoring protocols must be implemented, as well as the organization of a 24/7 vigilant and functional experienced RRT. This implies a significant financial investment to provide an only sporadically required fast intervention and sustained alertness of the people involved.

Keywords: early warning score, rapid response team, in-hospital cardiac arrest, proactive rounding

1. Introduction

While the organization and optimization of resuscitation of in-hospital cardiorespiratory collapse already receives due attention, there is a growing consciousness that a more

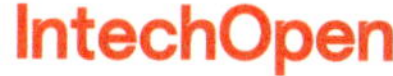

proactive strategy by improved detection of deteriorating patients and adequate intervention may prevent many inpatient deaths. This awareness is reflected in the 5 Million Lives campaign [1].

In the UK, the incidence of in-hospital cardiac arrest is 1.6/1000 hospital admissions [2]. Still, between 25 and 67% of the successfully in-hospital resuscitated patients die during the first 24 h after the return of spontaneous circulation (ROSC) [3]. In comparison, the survival to discharge after in-hospital cardiopulmonary resuscitation for cardiac arrest in nonelderly (18–64 years) in the US (2007–2012) was reported as only 30.4% and for patients >18 years as 27.4% [4, 5].

Particularly, in-hospital cardiorespiratory collapse is more frequently caused by preventable or correctable factors like respiratory problems or sepsis, compared to prehospital cardiorespiratory collapse, which is more frequently preceded by sudden, unexpected causes like cardiac rhythm disturbances or trauma [6].

In general, patients admitted to the intensive care unit (ICU) from hospital wards have a higher mortality risk compared to patients from theaters, postoperative recovery, or the emergency department. As such, there should be a focus on hospital wards to recognize patients who are critically ill prior to cardiopulmonary collapse [7].

Several studies have identified physiological abnormalities as a marker for clinical deterioration. Kause et al. [8] identified threatened airway, respiratory rate < 5, respiratory rate > 36, pulse rate < 40, pulse rate > 140, systolic blood pressure < 90 mmHg, fall of GCS by two points or more, and prolonged seizure activity. Goldhill et al. [9] defined the level of consciousness, heart rate, age, systolic pressure, and respiratory rate as predictive markers.

Based on a combination of those parameters, multiple scoring systems to identify patients at risk have been conceived, but they often lack validation [10].

Experience teaches that an exclusive implementation of a cardiac arrest team is both ineffective and expensive [7]. Keeping such a team continuously operational requires a significant financial investment [11], and the outcome remains poor [12]. Likewise, even advanced detection strategies, based on scoring systems to identify deteriorating patients, produced disappointing results [13]. This might be owing to a lack of validation of the scoring system [14]. In the MERIT study, a medical emergency team was implemented in 12 hospitals, and the outcome was compared with 11 other hospitals without such a team. The implementation of the team "greatly increased emergency team calling, but did not substantially affect the incidence of cardiac arrest, unplanned ICU admissions, or unexpected death". In this study, a rapid response team was implemented but still with disappointing results, which may be due to the lack of a reliable early warning system [12].

Above all, both afferent and efferent components are needed to be effective: a track-and-trigger system must be organized to firstly detect deteriorating patients early with suitable sensitivity and specificity, followed by a fast intervention by a professional team to optimize the treatment or bring the patient to an intensive care unit.

The managerial task for enabling such an effective program is, therefore, the implementation of reliable early identification of patient deterioration, followed by a fast and appropriate response without significantly increasing nurse workload and without turning ward areas into ICUs [15]. It consists of two separate systems working in tandem: an early warning system and a rapid response team.

Repetitive nursing staff education must provide fast and reliable patient scoring with high sensitivity and acceptable specificity. Secondly, to permit swift intervention when necessary, a dedicated hospital informatics system is required enabling the RRT to view all the patients in the hospital. Thirdly, detection of a deteriorating patient must prompt swift intervention.

2. The EWS scoring system

The British National Institute for Health and Clinical Excellence documented in the National Institute of Health and Clinical Excellence (NICE) 2007 guidelines [16] that physiological track and trigger systems should be used to monitor all adult patients and facilitate the recognition of patient deterioration. According to the scoring (low, medium, or high score group), a graded response strategy should be followed (**Figure 1**). A score is given to different

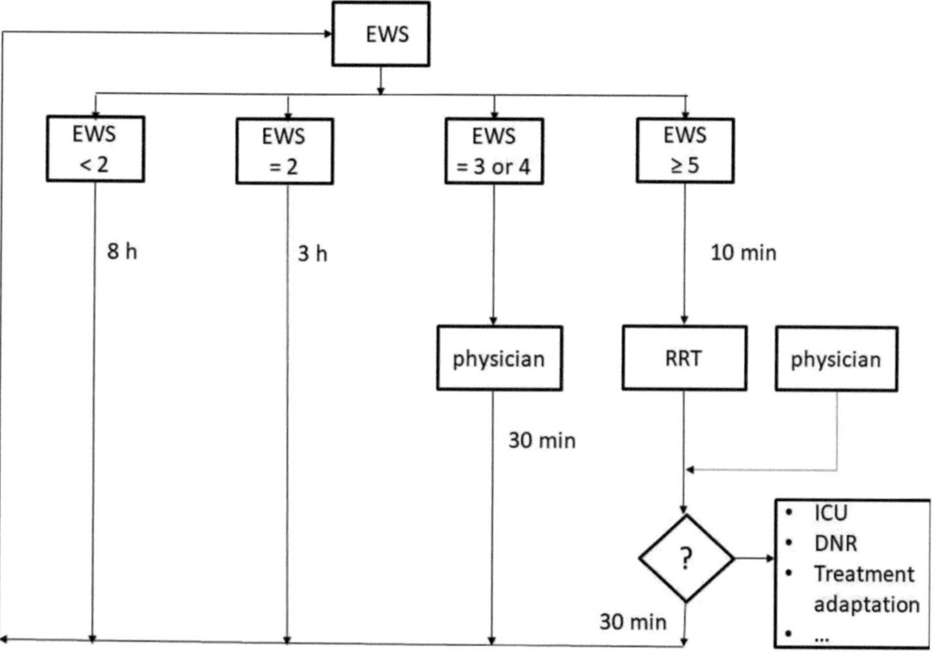

Figure 1. Example of a formalized decision process with graded response.

physiological measurements, which are often already routinely measured and recorded in hospitals. The magnitude of the score reflects how extreme the parameter deviates from the norm. The different scores are aggregated and uplifted for people requiring oxygen [17]. Depending on each calculated score, the algorithm provides a recommendation. At moderate scores, the frequency of subsequent clinical monitoring is increased to enable accelerated detection of deterioration. At higher scores, an increasingly urgent clinical assessment up to emergency intervention is triggered [17].

In the past, several scoring systems were proposed, where the weight allocated to each parameter defines the sensitivity of the final score to trigger a response. An expert working group reviewed the weightings used in a number of early warning score (EWS) systems such as the VitalPAC early warning score (ViEWS) [18] and made small adjustments based on the clinical opinion from the working group [17]. Different approaches can be proposed with divergent consideration and often conflicting priorities. In clinical practice, a scoring system needs to be integrated into daily practice and should, therefore, be user friendly and not too complex. Failure to meet this requirement will result in noncompliance and unreliable scoring. As such, the features of a system aiming for 100% sensitivity and specificity will differ from a convenient screening tool. The group also recommended a color-coded clinical chart to aid identification of abnormal clinical parameters.

2.1. Different parameters

Known statistically significant risk factors for cardiac arrest are as follows: abnormal respiratory rate, abnormal breathing, abnormal pulse, reduced systolic blood pressure, abnormal temperature, reduced pulse oximetry, chest pain, and nurse or doctor concern [19].

In addition, several clinical observations are significant predictors of mortality: decrease in Glasgow Coma score by two points, onset of coma, hypotension <90 mmHg, respiratory rate < 6/min, oxygen saturation < 90%, and bradycardia >30/min [20].

The National Institute for Health and Clinical Excellence (NICE) [16] and the National Early Warning Score (NEWS) Development and Implementation Group [17] recommended:

- Pulse rate

Tachycardia can reflect pyrexia, pain, general distress, cardiac arrhythmia, or circulatory compromise such as in sepsis, volume depletion, or cardiac failure. Bradycardia can be induced by medication, hypothermia, central nervous system (CNS) depression, heart block, and hypothyroidism.

- Respiratory rate

The respiratory rate is frequently the first parameter to change in the advent of clinical deterioration. Tachypnea can be induced by pain, distress, sepsis, CNS disturbance, and metabolic disturbance. Bradypnea can be due to CNS depression or narcosis [21]. Respiratory deterioration is one of the most common reasons for ICU admission. Early identification and treatment of these patients may, therefore, reduce ICU admission. Increased risk factors are chronic respiratory disease, sedation outside the operating room, and administration of patients who receive opioids [15]. The respiratory rate is elevated significantly above normal in a majority of patients with cardiac arrest [22] and is predictive of cardiac arrest [23].

- Systolic blood pressure

Hypertension can be a manifestation of cardiovascular disease or be a consequence of pain. Hypotension can be due to rhythm disturbance, CNS depression or naturally low blood pressure, or can reflect circulatory compromise such as sepsis, volume depletion, or cardiac failure. Hypotension is more indicative of acute illness than hypertension. Importantly, a change of systolic blood pressure was identified as an independent predictor of cardiac arrest [19], although earlier reports had concluded the opposite [23].

- Level of consciousness

This is quantified by alert-reaction to voice-reaction to pain-unresponsive (AVPU). This score is assessed in sequence and records only one outcome. Agitation also counts as an independent scoring point. Confusion is not part of the AVPU assessment, but recently developed confusion or worsening of confusion is a major concern and must trigger urgent clinical evaluation. Consciousness just failed statistical significance to predict cardiac arrest but was considered clinically significant, and therefore it was incorporated into the activation criteria [19]. Moreover, prior research had shown that 42% of the patients with cardiac arrest had alterations in mental function [22].

- Oxygen saturation

This is not always incorporated in the scores owing to the necessity for additional hardware. Pulse oximetry, however, is noninvasive and permits a rapid indication of oxygen levels but may be misleading due to false positive alarms. Pattern recognition of the waveform may improve the accuracy of these measurements [15]. Pulse oximetry cannot replace measurement of the respiratory rate [19], for which capnography is sometimes put forward as an alternative.

- Temperature, as a measure of pyrexia or hypothermia
- The requirement of supplemental oxygen for patients, which includes routine oxygen delivery by mask or nasal cannula. If present, a weighting score of two should be added, because patients are at greater clinical risk.

In a model reported in 2005, aiming to predict the need for intervention, all physiological components except temperature contributed significantly. Additionally, in the model predicting hospital outcome, all components except temperature and heart rate contributed [24]. Moreover, a higher number of events experienced by a patient were correlated with a higher risk of mortality [20].

In addition to the components included in the National Early Warning Score of the UK (NEWS), several variables are known risk factors for patient deterioration. The mortality increases significantly with age, although including age in the model offers little practical benefit in this context [18, 23, 25]. The urine output is essential for some patients, but it is not available at first assessment and is not routinely performed. It is recommended that it should only be assessed when clinically appropriate [16, 17]. Pain scores are included in the chart in NEWS but are not part of the aggregated scoring system.

Gender, ethnicity, and obesity alter several values, but this is not considered in most scoring systems. Likewise, during pregnancy, most parameters are modified. Conventional EWS triggers are therefore inapplicable in patients who are pregnant [17]. Several variables and comorbidities are for now not included in the EWS but may improve the model upon improved modeling. Abdominal pain, for instance, is not considered statistically significant in general but may be relevant in specific subpopulations [19]. Likewise, immunosuppression or other conditions may require disease-specific scoring systems. In addition, the inclusion of routine laboratory tests does not add sufficient consistency to be included in current EWS models [22], but advances in hospital informatics may change this in the future.

2.2. Scoring algorithms

The modified early warning score [26] prescribes a minimum frequency of monitoring of 12 h unless a decision has been made at a senior level to increase or decrease this frequency for an adult patient [17, 27]. If abnormal values are detected, the frequency of monitoring should increase [16]. The threshold should regularly be reviewed to optimize sensitivity and specificity [16]. Several strategies were explored to trigger the response [16]:

- Single-parameter system:

  This consists of periodic observations of selected vital signs that are compared with a simple set of criteria with predefined thresholds, with a response algorithm being activated when any of the criteria are met [20, 28]. Advantages of such a system are its ease of use and reproducibility. A significant disadvantage is that it permits only limited grade response strategy, and has low sensitivity, resulting in a lot of false negatives.

- Multiparameter system

  This response algorithm requires more than one criterion to be met, or the response differs according to the number of criteria met [9, 24]. This strategy allows monitoring and graded response strategy and has a higher sensitivity [29] but is expensive—owing to increased clinical contact time and additional equipment—and has low specificity when only one abnormal observation is present.

- Aggregate scoring system

  Weighted scores are assigned to physiological values and compared with predefined trigger thresholds [19, 26, 30]. Since this permits simple monitoring and a graded response strategy, it is widely used. It is however also expensive and is prone to human errors. The specificity and sensitivity depend on the used cut-off value.

- Combination system:

  This strategy is defined as multiple parameter systems used in combination with aggregate weighted scoring systems.

http://dx.doi.org/10.5772/intechopen.79651

While more time-consuming, an aggregate weighted scoring system is more sensitive than single parameter systems and therefore promoted in most guidelines [29].

2.3. Specific EWS systems

Clusters of hospitals often use the same scoring system. For instance, the patient-at-risk score (PARS) [24] is used in all hospitals of the Worcestershire Mental Help Partnership Trust. It facilitates patient and staff transfer between hospitals within the Trust. A particular purpose of nation-wide standardized systems, such as NEWS in the UK, is to avoid a lack of familiarity with local systems.

Importantly, NEWS cannot be used in children, pregnant women, or patients with chronically disturbed physiology, for example, chronic obstructive pulmonary disease (COPD), for which alternative systems are needed [17]. Such specific scoring systems are proposed for patients with chronic respiratory disease (e.g., CREWS – S-NEWS [31], sequential sepsis-related organ failure assessment [qSOFA]), and systemic inflammatory response syndrome [SIRS]) or in patients with suspected sepsis [32]. Implementation of a proposed pediatric scoring system (Bedside PEWS) however did not result in reduced mortality [33]. A specific neonatal trigger score (Neonati), however, showed better than PEWS [34].

2.4. Hospital informatics

To optimize the effectiveness of the RRT, particularly in case of automated recordings, the informatics system of the hospital should provide an electronic dashboard showing all hospital patients in a single view, ranked by EWS score and updated in real time. This permits immediate notification of deviant scores and swift intervention. Such a display also allows the RRT to take a proactive approach to see patients, monitor patients and review patients at risk, rather than relying exclusively on bedside nurses to activate the RRT. Until further research, the clinical benefit of an electronic dashboard remains unproven [35]. Nevertheless, it has a very promising advantage that it permits an active search for the patients who are the most at risk in the hospital. This allows the RRT to visit and eventually treat the patients in the ward proactively. In addition, the electronic dashboard can also be considered an approach to reduce alert fatigue in the RRT.

2.5. EWS scoring as standard-of-care

Of particular importance for optimal performance is the managerial endorsement that the EWS assessments and consequential RRT interventions are a hospital-wide standard-of-care protocol. As such, all measurements are standardized nursing measures for which no permission or instruction of the physician is required. Only individualized opting-out is possible, but this must be prescribed for each individual patient as a written medical order if deemed suitable.

2.6. DNR registration

In patients with a do not resuscitate (DNR) code higher than 3, the RRT will not be mobilized. Still, also when the RRT is mobilized, they will consider the DNR code in further patient management. The awareness of the importance of the DNR code on the RRT interventions will often also result in its more correct and timely registration. The subsequently improved decision-making regarding patient suitability for DNR orders can be one of the explanations of reduced incidence of resuscitations in several reports [29].

3. The rapid response team

3.1. Organization of the response

After reliable identification of patients at risk, the efferent component of the system must be initiated as fast as possible. The first report about the institution of RRTs is dated from 1995 [36]. Initially, in-hospital interventions were also assigned to the regular medical emergency team, but soon specific teams were "tailored to the specific population it serves" [29].

Likewise, the decision to mobilize the RRT was initially left to the personal assessment of the nurse, but in subsequent improvements, the decision-making process was increasingly formalized. An example of such a formalized decision process is shown in **Figure 1**.

3.2. Composition of the team

The composition of the current teams varies between different countries and care systems [8, 29]. Of utmost importance, effective inter-professional communication between and among nurses and doctors is essential for an adequate response [37]. There is still discussion about whether a physician should be part of the RRT, and a meta-analysis did not identify the presence of a physician to be significantly associated with mortality reduction [38]. In addition, the effect of the presence of a physician might be different in university hospitals versus community hospitals, and the response to deterioration might be most effective when a clinician leads it [29]. A recent comprehensive review concluded that there is evidence that RRTs are effective in reducing readmission to ICU (2+) and in reducing hospital mortality (2+) [29].

Hospitalist physicians have been integrated on the general wards in US hospitals since 1996 [39] and might be useful members of the rapid response team. These hospitalists are mostly specialized in general internal medicine and have a coordinating function with a focus on the general medical care of hospitalized patients [40]. Not only are they an important information pool for patients, family members, nurses, and consultants, they also can assign additional diagnostic and therapeutic activities in case of urgent situations [40]. A positive effect of the introduction of hospitalists on the patients' average length of hospital stay and total hospital costs has already been demonstrated [39] but seems to be dependent on the hospitalist workload [41]. Including a hospital physician in the rapid response team can immediately increase the knowledge of a specific patient and decrease the code call rate. However, it does not seem to affect the general hospital mortality rate [42].

Recently, it is believed that there is a need for an acute care physician or so-called resuscitationist who cooperates with specialized trauma surgeons [43]. Currently, there is no data present which evaluate the effect of the resuscitationist on the outcome of the patient population [44]. Since these physicians are specialized in resuscitation, trauma, and critically ill and emergency patients [44] they might have essential skills to participate in the RRT.

Similar to other physicians, both the acute care physician and hospitalist can bring valuable knowledge to the RRT but are often not able to prioritize RRT calls due to additional tasks and a usually high workload. In practice, a specialized nurse-driven team is therefore often necessary to guarantee an immediate RRT response, while close communication and cooperation with specialized physicians are expected to improve the decision-making process.

3.3. Organization of 24/7 availability

Because of the significant financial cost of a 24/7 operational RRT, while the team is not performing interventions most of the time, they are often attributed other responsibilities within the hospital. It is however imperative that absolute priority is given to the necessary monitoring and interventions to preserve its full effect. When the RRT is not operational 100% of the time, there exists a significant risk that during the absence of the trained RRT, its responsibilities are passed back on the most inexperienced members of the clinical team [29]. Following the NEWS guidelines, the RRT should be free of other clinical responsibilities and available 24/7 [17].

3.4. Educational component

In addition to the implementation of the EWS and RRT, a strong and sustained educational component is of vital importance toward both reducing cardiac arrests and improving decision-making [29]. Recent studies have shown that for an RRT to be successful, it must be implemented with a continuing medical education program [45]. A nurse-driven approach often lowers the threshold for effective communication, improving the educational effect on the nursing staff, ultimately leading to more accurate detection of patient deterioration.

4. Impact of EWS-RRT implementation

The impact of EWS-RRT implementation has been extensively described and resumed in a comprehensive review [29]. Beneficial effects have been shown for specific outcomes, but a comparison is difficult owing to heterogeneities, including but not limited to study design, team composition, duration, RRT area, and nomenclature [38]. As such, standardized reporting is needed to enable comparative analysis [46]. Decreases have been reported in the incidence of cardiac arrest [47–50] and in cardiac arrest mortality [49, 51]. A reported decrease in in-hospital mortality of 1580 lives in the study population would extrapolate to over 100,000 lives saved in Western Europe [50, 52].

The economic implications of an implementation are difficult to measure [11], as the cost of the monitoring outreach team and additional costs at ward level, the use of equipment, and clinical contact time must be compared to the reduction in ICU admissions/readmissions [16].

An unexpected additional advantage may be a more accurate registration of the DNR code [50]. As the RRT improves the quality of care via early identification/reversal of physiological decompensation, this may lead to a more timely activation of palliative therapies and as such enhanced end-of-life care [53].

5. Pitfalls during the implementation

The response of the RRT may suffer from excessive false alerts, making the team desensitized, leading to alarm fatigue [15, 38, 54]. This underlines the necessity of a scoring system with sufficient specificity, such as an aggregate score like EWS.

Manual registration of some variables, such as the respiratory rate, might incite the recording of inaccurate values to limit subsequent burden. Moreover, it is generally recommended that the respiratory rate be counted over a whole minute or two 30 s intervals, and this procedure can represent a significant investment in nursing time in the ward setting, such that accurate rates may only be recorded as little as 37% of the time [15]. The respiratory rate is therefore often particularly poorly recorded, although it may be the most important early manifestation of critical illness [7, 21]. The long-term effectiveness of the program may also decrease in the absence of periodic training and therefore requires continued educational investment [51].

6. Conclusions

The prevention of in-hospital resuscitations requires a "whole system" approach, consisting of a reliable EWS, combined with an effective RRT, sustained feedback, and focused education. In addition to the implementation of the dedicated systems and teams, its effectiveness necessitates a changing culture of the whole organization.

Conflict of interest

No conflicts of interest.

Author details

Alain Kalmar*, Nicky Van Der Vekens, Henk Vanoverschelde, Diederik Van Sassenbroeck, Jan Heerman and Tom Verbeke

*Address all correspondence to: alain.kalmar@azmmsj.be

Department of Anesthesia and Critical Care Medicine, Maria Middelares Hospital, Ghent, Belgium

References

[1] Lewis C. 5 Million lives campaign. Journal of Vascular Nursing. 2007;**25**(3):57. DOI: 10.1016/j.jvn.2007.06.007

[2] Nolan JP, Soar J, Smith GB, Gwinnutt C, Parrot F, Power S, et al. Incidence and outcome of in-hospital cardiac arrest in the United Kingdom National Cardiac Arrest Audit. Resuscitation. 2014;**85**(8):987-992. DOI: 10.1016/j.resuscitation.2014.04.002

[3] Sandroni C, Nolan J, Cavallaro F, Antonelli M. In-hospital cardiac arrest: Incidence, prognosis and possible measures to improve survival. Intensive Care Medicine. 2007;**33**(2): 237-245. DOI: 10.1007/s00134-006-0326-z

[4] Mallikethi-Reddy S, Briasoulis A, Akintoye E, Jagadeesh K, Brook RD, Rubenfire M, et al. Incidence and survival after in-hospital cardiopulmonary resuscitation in noneldery adults: US experience, 2007 to 2012. Circulation: Cardiovascular Quality and Outcomes. 2017;**10**(2):e003194. DOI: 10.1161/circoutcomes.116.003194

[5] Kolte D, Khera S, Aronow WS, Palaniswamy C, Mujib M, Ahn C, et al. Regional variation in the incidence and outcomes of in-hospital cardiac arrest in the United States. Circulation. 2015;**131**(16):1415-1425. DOI: 10.1161/circulationaha.114.014542

[6] Monteleone PP, Lin CM. In-hospital cardiac arrest. Emergency Medicine Clinics of North America. 2012;**30**(1):25-34. DOI: 10.1016/j.emc.2011.09.005

[7] Goldhill DR. The critically ill: following your MEWS. QJM. 2001;**94**(10):507-510. DOI: 10.1093/qjmed/94.10.507

[8] Kause J, Smith G, Prytherch D, Parr M, Flabouris A, Hillman K. A comparison of antecedents to cardiac arrests, deaths and emergency intensive care admissions in Australia and New Zealand, and the United Kingdom – The ACADEMIA study. Resuscitation. 2004;**62**(3):275-282. DOI: 10.1016/j.resuscitation.2004.05.016

[9] Goldhill DR, McNarry AF. Physiological abnormalities in early warning scores are related to mortality in adult inpatients. British Journal of Anaesthesia. 2004;**92**(6):882-884. DOI: 10.1093/bja/aeh113

[10] Smith GB, Prytherch DR, Schmidt PE, Featherstone PI. Review and performance evaluation of aggregate weighted 'track and trigger' systems. Resuscitation. 2008;**77**(2):170-179. DOI: 10.1016/j.resuscitation.2007.12.004

[11] Murphy A, Cronin J, Whelan R, Drummond FJ, Savage E, Hegarty J. Economics of early warning scores for identifying clinical deterioration – A systematic review. Irish Journal of Medical Science. 2018;**187**(1):193-205. DOI: 10.1007/s11845-017-1631-y

[12] Hillman K, Chen J, Cretikos M, Bellomo R, Brown D, Doig G, et al. MERIT study investigators. Introduction of the medical emergency team (MET) system: A cluster-randomised controlled trial. Lancet. 2005;**365**(9477):2091-2097. DOI: 10.1016/s0140-6736(05)66733-5

[13] Haegdorens F, Van Bogaert P, Roelant E, De Meester K, Misselyn M, Wouters K, et al. The introduction of a rapid response system in acute hospitals: A pragmatic stepped wedge cluster randomised controlled trial. Resuscitation. 2018 Apr 18. [Epub ahead of print]. DOI: 10.1016/j.resuscitation.2018.04.018

[14] Gerry S, Birks J, Bonnici T, Watkinson PK, Kirtley S, Collins GS. Early warning scores for detecting deterioration in adult hospital patients: A systematic review protocol. BMJ Open. 2017;**7**(12):e019268. DOI: 10.1136/bmjopen-2017-019268

[15] Vincent JL, Einav S, Pearse R, Jaber S, Kranke P, Overdyk FJ, et al. Improving detection of patient deterioration in the general hospital ward environment. European Journal of Anaesthesiology. 2018;**35**(5):325-333. DOI: 10.1097/eja.0000000000000798

[16] National Institute for Health and Clinical Excellence (NICE). Acutely Ill Patients in Hospital: Recognition of and Response to Acute Illness in Adults in Hospital. NICE Clinical Guideline 50. London, United Kingdom; 2007

[17] Royal College of Physicians. National Early Warning Score (NEWS) 2: Standardising the Assessment of Acute-illness Severity in the NHS. Updated report of a working party. London, United Kingdom: RCP; 2017

[18] Prytherch DR, Smith GB, Schmidt PE, Feathersone PI. ViEWS–Towards a national early warning score for detecting adult inpatient deterioration. Resuscitation. 2010;**81**(8):932-937. DOI: 10.1016/j.resuscitation.2010.04.014

[19] Hodgetts TJ, Kenward G, Vlachonikolis IG, Payne S, Castle N. The identification of risk factors for cardiac arrest and formulation of activation criteria to alert a medical emergency team. Resuscitation. 2002;**54**(2):125-131. DOI: 10.1016/s0300-9572(02)00100-4

[20] Buist M, Bernard S, Nguyen TV, Moore G, Anderson J. Association between clinically abnormal observations and subsequent in-hospital mortality: a prospective study. Resuscitation. 2004;**62**(2):137-141. DOI: 10.1016/j.resuscitation.2004.03.005

[21] McBride J, Knight D, Piper J, Smith GB. Long-term effect of introducing an early warning score on respiratory rate charting on general wards. Resuscitation. 2005;**65**(1):41-44. DOI: 10.1016/j.resuscitation.2004.10.015

[22] Schein R, Hazday N, Pena M, Ruben B, Sprung CL. Clinical antecedents to in-hospital cardiopulmonary arrest. Chest. 1990;**98**(6):1388-1392. DOI: 10.1378/chest.98.6.1388

[23] Fieselmann JF, Hendryx SM, Helms CM, Wakefield DS. Respiratory rate predicts cardiopulmonary arrest for internal medicine inpatients. Journal of General Internal Medicine. 1993;**8**(7):354-360. DOI: 10.1007/bf02600071

[24] Goldhill DR, McNarry AF, Mandersloot G, McGinley A. A physiologically-based early warning score for ward patients: the association between score and outcome. Anaesthesia. 2005;**60**(6):547-553. DOI: 10.1111/j.1365-2044.2005.04186.x

[25] Royal College of Physicians. National Early Warning Score (NEWS): Standardising the Assessment of Acute-illness Severity in the NHS. Report of a working party. London, United Kingdom: RCP; 2012

[26] Subbe CP, Kruger M, Rutherford P, Gemmel L. Validation of a modified early warning score in medical admission. QJM: An International Journal of Medicine. 2001;**94**(10):521-526. DOI: 10.1093/qjmed/94.10.521

[27] Petersen JA, Antonsen K, Rasmussen LS. Frequency of early warning score assessment and clinical deterioration in hospitalized patients: A randomized trial. Resuscitation. 2016;**101**:91-96. DOI: 10.1016/j.resuscitation.2016.02.003

[28] Bell MB, Konrad D, Granath F, Ekbom A, Marling C-R. Prevalence and sensitivity of MET-criteria in a Scandinavian University Hospital. Resuscitation. 2006;**70**(1):66-73. DOI: 10.1016/j.resuscitation.2005.11.011

[29] McNeill G, Bryden D. Do either early warning systems or emergency response teams improve hospital patient survival? A systematic review. Resuscitation. 2013;**84**(12):1652-1667. DOI: 10.1016/j.resuscitation.2013.08.006

[30] Duckitt RW, Buxton-Thomas R, Walker J, Cheek E, Bewick V, Venn R, et al. Worthing physiological scoring system: derivation and validation of a physiological early-warning system for medical admissions. An observation, population-based single-centre study. British Journal of Anaesthesia. 2007;**98**(6):769-774. DOI: 10.1093/bja/aem097

[31] Pedersen NE, Rasmussen LS, Petersen JA, Gerds TA, Østergaard D, Lippert A. Modifications of the National early warning score for patients with chronic respiratory disease. Acta Anaesthesiologica Scandinavica. 2007;**62**(2):242-252. DOI: 10.1111/aas.13020

[32] Finkelsztein EJ, Jones DS, Ma KC, Pabón MA, Delgado T, Nakahira K, et al. Comparison of qSOFA and SIRS for predicting adverse outcomes of patients with suspicion of sepsis outside the intensive care unit. Critical Care. 2017;**21**(1):73-83. DOI: 10.1186/s13054-017-1658-5

[33] Parshuram CS, Dryden-Palmer K, Farrell C, Gottesman R, Gray M, Hutchinson J, et al. Effect of a pediatric early warning system on all-cause mortality in hospitalized pediatric patients. The EPOCH randomized clinical trial. JAMA. 2018;**319**(10):1002-1012. DOI: 10.1001/jama.2018.0948

[34] Holme H, Bhatt R, Koumettou M, Griffin MAS, Winckworth LC. Retrospective evaluation of a new Neonatal Trigger Score. Pediatrics. 2013;**131**(3):e837-e842. DOI: 10.1542/peds.2012-0640d

[35] Fletcher GS, Aaronson BA, White AA, Julka R. Effect of a real-time electronic dashboard on a rapid response system. Journal of Medical Systems. 2018;**42**(1):1-10. DOI: 10.4271/890106

[36] Lee A, Bishop G, Hillman KM, Daffurn K. The medical emergency team. Anaesthesia and Intensive Care. 1995;**23**(2):183-186

[37] De Meester K, Verspuy M, Monsieurs KG. SBAR improves nurse-physician communication and reduces unexpected death: A pre and post intervention study. Resuscitation. 2013;**84**(9):1192-1196. DOI: 10.1016/j.resuscitation.2013.03.016

[38] Maharaj R, Raffaele I, Wendon J. Rapid response systems: A systematic review and meta-analysis. Critical Care. 2015;**19**(1):254-269. DOI: 10.1186/s13054-015-0973-y

[39] White HL, Glazier RH. Do hospitalist physicians improve the quality of inpatient care delivery? A systematic review of process, efficiency and outcome measures. BMC Medicine. 2011;**18**(9):58. DOI: 10.1186/1741-7015-9-58

[40] Burkhardt U, Erbsen A, Rüdger-Stürchler M. The hospitalist as coordinator: An observational case study. Journal of Health Organization and Management. 2010;**24**(1):22-44. DOI: 10.1108/14777261011029552

[41] Elliot DJ, Young RS, Brice J, Aguiar R, Kolm P. Effect of hospitalist workload on the quality and efficiency of care. JAMA Internal Medicine. 2014;**174**(5):786-793. DOI: 10.1001/jamainternmed.2014.300

[42] Rothberg MB, Belforti R, Fitzgerald J, Friderici J, Keyes M. Four years' experience with a hospitalist-led medical emergency team: An interrupted time series. Journal of Hospital Medicine. 2012;**7**(2):98-103. DOI: 10.1002/jhm.953

[43] Conti B, Greco KM, McCunn M. The acute care anesthesiologist as resuscitationist. International Anesthesiology Clinics. 2017;**55**(3):109-116. DOI: 10.1097/AIA.0000000000000148

[44] McCunn M, Dutton RP, Dagal A, Varon AJ, Kaslow O, Kucik CJ, et al. Trauma, critical care, and emergency care anesthesiology: a new paradigm for the "acute care" anesthesiologist? Anesthesia and Analgesia. 2015;**121**(6):1668-1673. DOI: 10.1213/ANE.0000000000000782

[45] Calzavacca P, Licari E, Tee A, Egi M, Downey A, Quach J, et al. The impact of Rapid Response System on delayed emergency team activation patient characteristics and outcomes–A follow-up study. Resuscitation. 2010;**81**(1):31-35. DOI: 10.1016/j.resuscitation.2009.09.026

[46] Peberdy MA, Cretikos M, Abella BS, DeVita M, Goldhill D, Kloeck W, et al. Recommended guidelines for monitoring, reporting and conducting research on medical emergency team, outreach and rapid response systems: An Utstein-style scientific statement. A scientific statement from the international Liaison committee on resuscitation; the American Heart Association Emergency Cardiovascular Care Committee; the Council on Cardiopulmonary, Perioperative, and Critical Care; and the Interdisciplinary Working Group on Quality of Care and Outcomes Research. Resuscitation. 2007;**75**(21):412-433. DOI: 10.1016/j.resuscitation.2007.09.009

[47] Buist M, Harrison J, Abaloz E, Van Dyke S, Harrison R. Quality improvement report: Six year audit of cardiac arrests and medical emergency team calls in an Australian outer metropolitan teaching hospital. British Medical Journal. 2007;**335**(7631):1210-1212. DOI: 10.1136/bmj.39385.534236.47

[48] Buist MD, Moore GE, Bernard SE, Waxman BP, Anderson JN, Nguyen TV. Effects of a medical emergency team on reduction of incidence of and mortality from unexpected cardiac arrests in hospital: Preliminary study. British Medical Journal. 2002;**324**(7334):387-390. DOI: 10.1136/bmj.324.7334.387

[49] Davis DP, Graham PG, Husa RD, Lawrence B, Minokadeh A, Altieri K, et al. A performance improvement-based resuscitation programme reduces arrest incidence and

increases survival from in-hospital cardiac arrest. Resuscitation. 2015;**95**:63-69. DOI: 10.1016/j.resuscitation.2015.04.008

[50] Chen J, Ou L, Flabouris A, Hillman K, Bellomo R, Parr M. Impact of a standardized rapid response system on outcomes in a large healthcare jurisdiction. Resuscitation. 2016;**107**: 47-56. DOI: 10.1016/j.resuscitation.2016.07.240

[51] Campello G, Granja C, Carvalho F, Dias C, Azevedo L-F, Costa-Pereira A. Immediate and long-term Impact of medical emergency teams on cardiac arrests prevalence and mortality: A plea for periodic basis life-support training programs. Critical Care Medicine. 2009;**37**(12):3054-3061. DOI: 10.1097/CCM.0b013e3181b02183

[52] De Jong A, Jung B, Daurat A, Chanques G, Mahul M, Monnin M, et al. Effect of rapid response systems on hospital mortality: A systematic review and meta-analysis. 2016;**42**(4):615-617. DOI: 10.1007/s00134-016-4263-1

[53] Vasquez R, Gheorghe C, Grigoriyan A, Palvinskaya T, Amoateng-Adjepong Y, Manthous CA. Enhanced end-of-life care associated with deploying a Rapid Response Team: A pilot study. Journal of Hospital Medicine. 2009;**4**(7):449-452. DOI: 10.1002/jhm.451

[54] Jones D, Bellomo R, Devita AM. Effectiveness of the medical emergency team: The importance of dose. Critical Care. 2009;**13**(5):313. DOI: 10.1186/cc7996

Chapter 3

Resuscitation of Term Infants in the Delivery Room

Francesca Viaroli and Georg M. Schmölzer

Additional information is available at the end of the chapter

http://dx.doi.org/10.5772/intechopen.79394

Abstract

The majority of newborn infants make the transition from fetal-to-neonatal live without help. However, around 20% of newborn infants fail to initiate breathing at birth. In these cases, the clinical team has to provide respiratory support, which remains the cornerstone of neonatal resuscitation. This chapter will discuss respiratory support during neonatal resuscitation in both term and preterm infants. The chapter will discuss the respiratory fetal-to-neonatal transition, use of oxygen, mask ventilation and their pitfalls, the application of sustained inflation, positive end expiratory pressure, continuous positive airway pressures, and whether extremely low birth weight infants should be intubated immediately after birth or supported noninvasively.

Keywords: delivery room, resuscitation, newborn, infants

1. Introduction

Before birth, the fetus uses the placenta for gas exchange; however, immediately after birth, the infants has to clear lung liquid fluid and replace it with air, start spontaneous breathing, establish a functional residual capacity (FRC) in order to achieve gas exchange [1–3]. Approximately 85% of babies born at term will initiate spontaneous respirations within 10 to 30 seconds of birth, an additional 10% will respond during drying and stimulation, approximately 3% will initiate respirations after PPV, 2% will be intubated to support respiratory function, and 0.1% will require CC and/or epinephrine to achieve this transition [4–6]. When newborns fail to initiate spontaneous breathing, the International Liaison Committee on Resuscitation (ILCOR) recommend several steps to support the transition of newborn infants [4–6]. The initial steps of stabilization algorithm include providing warmth to maintain a normal body temperature by *drying* the infant, clearing any secretion if needed by using *suction*, and *stimulating* the infant to initiate breathing [4–6]. If these steps are unsuccessful, the clinical

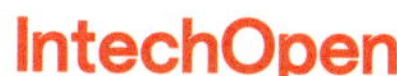

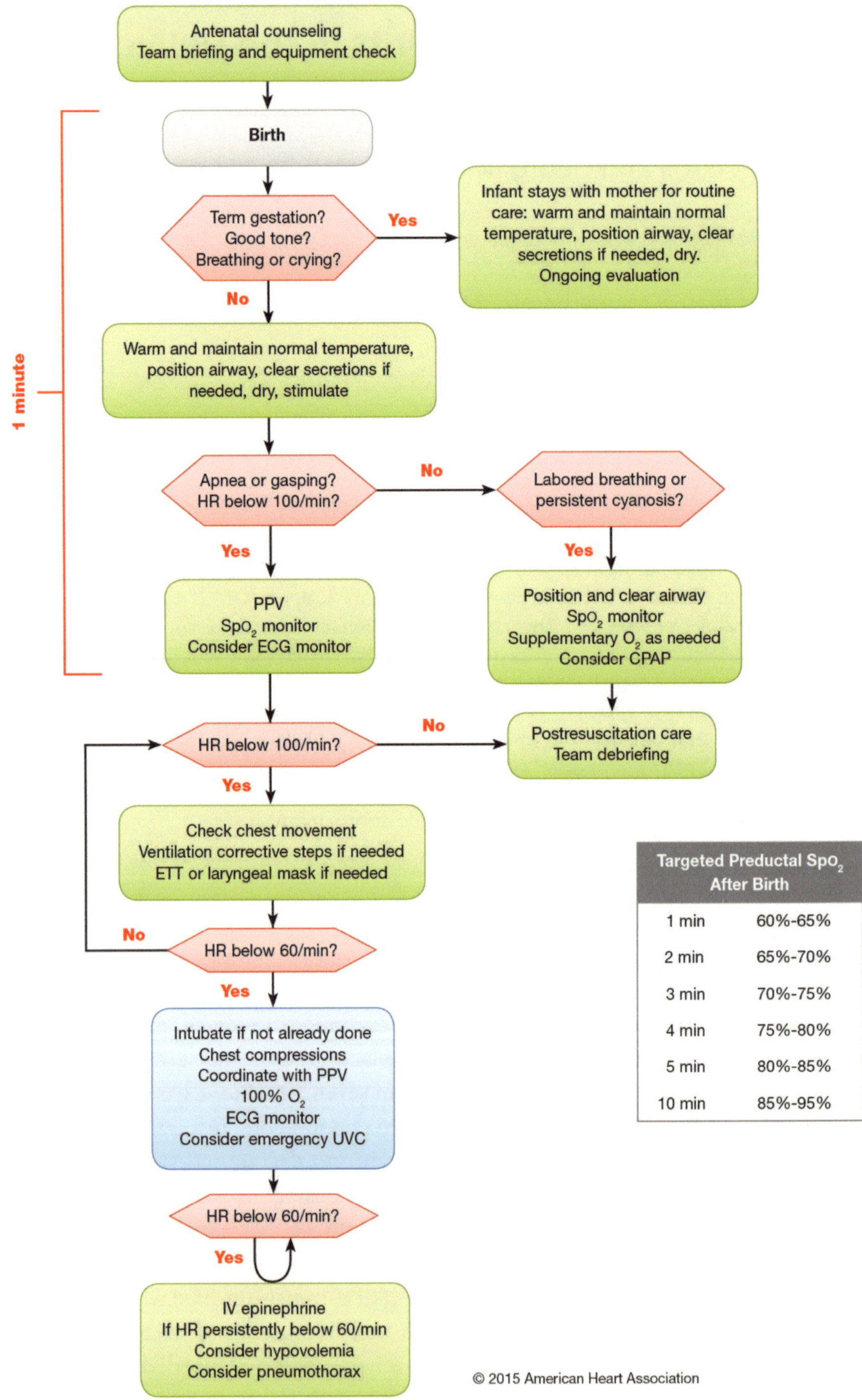

Figure 1. NRP algorithm.

team must initiate *mask positive pressure ventilation* (PPV) using a face mask and a ventilation device [4–6]. Adequate ventilation is the cornerstone of successful neonatal resuscitation; therefore, it is mandatory that anybody involved in neonatal resuscitation is trained in mask ventilation techniques [4–6]. In the rare cases (0.1% in term infants) where mask PPV is unsuccessful, more extensive resuscitation measures (*chest compression* (CC) and *epinephrine*) are needed (**Figure 1**) [4–6]. This chapter will discuss these various steps during stabilization/resuscitation of term infants in the delivery room (DR).

2. Initial steps of stabilization (drying, suction, and stimulation)

The initial steps of newborn stabilization/resuscitation are to maintain normal temperature of the infant, position the infant in a "sniffing" position to open the airway, clear secretions if needed with a bulb syringe or suction catheter, dry the infant, and stimulate the infant [4–6]. Most newborn infants are breathing or crying and have good tone immediately after birth [7, 8]. However, they must be dried and kept warm to avoid hypothermia, which can happen while the baby is lying on the mother's chest to avoid separation of mother and baby [4–6]. Maintaining normal temperature after birth is crucial due to a dose-dependent increase in mortality for temperatures <36.5°C [9]. Simple interventions (e.g., skin-to-skin contact or kangaroo mother care, plastic wrap, radiant warmer, thermal mattress, or warmed humidified resuscitation gases) to prevent hypothermia during transition (birth until 1 to 2 hours of life) can reduce mortality [4–6, 10, 11]. Maternal hyperthermia in labor is associated with adverse neonatal effects including increased mortality, neonatal seizures, and adverse neurologic states like encephalopathy [4–6]. Similarly, neonatal hyperthermia >38.0°C should be avoided due to the potential associated risks [4–6].

Suctioning immediately after birth, whether with a bulb syringe or suction catheter, should only be done if the airway appears obstructed or if PPV is required [4–6]. Avoiding unnecessary suctioning helps prevent the risk of induced bradycardia due to suctioning of the nasopharynx [4–6]. The presence of meconium-stained amniotic fluid may indicate fetal distress and increases the risk that the infant will require resuscitation after birth; therefore, a team that includes an individual skilled in tracheal intubation should be present at the time of birth [4–6]. Any infant who is vigorous with good respiratory effort and muscle tone may stay with their mother to receive the initial steps of newborn care [4–6]. Any infant presenting with poor muscle tone and inadequate breathing efforts after being born through meconium-stained amniotic fluid should receive the initial steps of resuscitation under a radiant warmer [4–6]. PPV should be initiated if the infant is not breathing or the heart rate is less than 100/min after the initial steps are completed [4–6]. Routine intubation for tracheal suction in this setting is not suggested, because there is insufficient evidence to continue recommending this practice [4–6].

Tactile stimulation including warming, drying, and rubbing the back or the soles of the feet is recommended in the current ILCOR guidelines [4–6]. Tactile stimulation is the first step to stimulate spontaneous breathing in newborn infants [4–6]. Retrospective studies reported a large variability in the use of tactile stimulation during the stabilization of infants at birth [12].

Furthermore, a recent randomized trial reported an increase in respiratory effort during repetitive stimulation compared to standard tactile stimulation with less oxygen requirements during transport to the NICU [13]. However, it did not reach significance, and further studies are needed.

2.1. Oxygen delivery during stabilization/resuscitation

The fetal oxygen saturation before birth is between 40 and 60% [14], which increases in uncompromised term infants within the first 10 minutes following birth to levels between 90 and 100% [15], thus resulting in the appearance of cyanosis during that time [16]. In addition, clinical assessment of skin color or the lack of cyanosis is a very poor indicator of oxygen saturation during that period [16–19]. The optimal management of oxygen during neonatal resuscitation becomes particularly important because of the evidence that either insufficient or excessive oxygenation can be harmful to the term infant with hypoxia and ischemia are known to result in injury to multiple organs and hyperoxia causing increased mortality [16, 20, 21]. Therefore, infants >35 weeks' gestation should be resuscitated in 21% oxygen and oxygen should be increased only if heart rate does not increase despite adequate ventilation.

3. Mask ventilation

Approximately, 10% of newborns require respiratory support at birth [22]. ILCOR and various national guidelines recommend techniques and equipment for neonatal resuscitation [4–6]. They all agree that mask ventilation is the cornerstone of respiratory support immediately after birth [4–6]. The purpose of PPV is to establish FRC, deliver an adequate V_T to facilitate gas exchange, and stimulate breathing while minimizing lung injury [2]. Several factors can reduce the effectiveness of mask ventilation, including poor face mask technique resulting in leak or airway obstruction, spontaneous movements of the baby, movements by or distraction of the resuscitator, and procedures such as changing the wraps or fitting a hat [23, 24]. Delivery room studies have shown that mask PPV is difficult, and mask leak and airway obstruction are common [23–29]. Both leak and obstruction are usually unrecognized unless expired CO_2 detectors or respiratory function monitors (RFM) are used [23–29]. In addition, airway maneuvers (e.g., jaw thrust or chin lift) to maintain airway patency is a crucial step during mask PPV [30].

4. Ventilation devices during respiratory support in the delivery room

There is currently limited evidence to guide clinicians' choice of the device to be used to provide PPV in the DR [31]. Self-inflating bags, flow-inflating bags, or T-piece devices may all be used for mask PPV [4–6]. A self-inflating bag, however, does not provide PEEP or continuous positive airway pressure (CPAP) [32, 33]. An attached PEEP-valve provides inconsistent

PEEP and cannot deliver CPAP [32–37]. A flow-inflating bag provides variable and operator dependent PEEP [16, 38]. With a T-piece device more consistent, predetermined levels of PEEP and PIP can be delivered [34, 35]. In addition, a T-piece device has been shown to be the most accurate device for delivering a sustained inflation [35, 39–41].

5. Interfaces

5.1. Face mask and nasal prongs

Effective and consistent PPV is important to facilitate lung aeration, establishment of a functional residual capacity, and gas exchange, which should occur in a predictable manner so that the clinician can avoid under- or over-inflating the lungs [2, 42–44]. However, PPV is often complicated by mask leak or airway obstruction [23–29]. Currently, clinicians can either use a face mask or a nasal prong during mask PPV [4–6]; however, face mask ventilation remains the primary mode of resuscitation. There are a variety of face masks available to provide PPV [25, 45, 46]. The Fisher & Paykel (F&P) (Fisher & Paykel Healthcare, Auckland, New Zealand) and the Laerdal round masks are the most commonly used commercially available products [47–52]. Although, face masks for preterm infants <33 weeks' do not adequately fit their face [53], the only study comparing F&P vs. Laerdal masks reported no difference in mask leak during PPV in the DR in preterm infants <33 weeks' [25]. Similarly, two studies compared face masks to nasal prongs in the DR and reported no difference in intubation in the delivery room [45, 46]. These data suggest that either face mask or nasal prong could be used for PPV in the DR and the focus should rather be on delivery of an adequate tidal volume to achieve lung aeration.

5.2. Laryngeal mask

Archie Brain, a British anesthetist, described the laryngeal mask airway (LMA) as an alternative to endotracheal intubation in 1981 [54]. A LMA consists of an airway tube connected distally to a soft elliptical mask with an inflatable rim to fit over the laryngeal inlet, whereas the proximal end connects to the ventilation device [54]. LMAs are routinely used in emergency and operating rooms for adult and pediatric anesthesia and ambulance services [55, 56]. In newborn infants, there is increasing evidence from randomized trials [57, 58], suggesting that a LMA can provide an effective rescue airway during resuscitation if both mask ventilation and endotracheal intubation have been unsuccessful. Current neonatal resuscitation guidelines recommend the use of LMA in infants >34 weeks' gestation or > 2000 g birth weight. Furthermore, LMA have been described during neonatal transport [59–61], provision of prolonged mechanical ventilation in particular for infants with upper airway abnormalities [62–64], and surfactant and epinephrine administration [65–69]. Although LMAs are recommended by various neonatal resuscitation guidelines, they are not routinely used during neonatal resuscitation [4–6].

5.3. Oropharyngeal airway

In 1907, Sir Fredrick Hewitt presented the first known artificial oral "air-way" to alleviate upper airway obstruction, a common problem during general anesthesia [31]. In 1933, Arthur Guedel presented "the Guedel oropharyngeal airway" [37], designed to hold the tongue away from the back of the pharynx, thus providing a clear channel for respired gases [70]. An oropharyngeal airways may be used to open the airway in floppy newborn infants, or if mask ventilation is ineffective [71–74]. In addition, various surveys evaluating neonatal resuscitation practice reported that Guedel airways are part of the neonatal resuscitation equipment [50, 75]. Guedel airways for newborn infants come in traditional sizes of 000, 00, and 0. However, oropharyngeal airways during neonatal resuscitation have not been systematically studied, and only one trial is currently ongoing comparing an oropharyngeal airway for prevention of airway obstruction during PPV in preterm infants <34 weeks' gestation in the DR [49]. Until further evidence is available, oropharyngeal airway should be used with caution.

6. Ventilation modes

When infants fail to initiate spontaneous breathing, the current neonatal resuscitation guidelines recommend mask PPV using any above described ventilation devices coupled with a face mask or a nasal prong [4–6]. The purpose of PPV is to establish FRC, deliver an adequate V_T to facilitate gas exchange, and stimulate breathing while minimizing lung injury [2]. The current neonatal resuscitation guidelines further recommend to use a peak inflation pressure of around 30 cm H_2O, a positive end expiratory pressure of 5 cm H_2O when using a T-Piece or a flow-inflating bag, and a gas flow rate of 10 L/min and 21% oxygen [4–6]. Oxygen should only be increased if the infant requires chest compression (see the paragraph below), the heart rate does not increase despite adequate ventilation, or if SpO_2 is below the recommend target range [4–6]. If infants have adequate spontaneous respiration, but remain cyanotic (e.g., SpO_2 is below the recommend target range [4–6]) during the initial stabilization, CPAP using pressures between 5 and 8 cm H_2O should be provided using a T-Piece or a flow-inflating bag (see the paragraph about ventilation devices).

There is no need for any other ventilation modalities (e.g., high frequency ventilation or mechanical ventilation) in the delivery room, which should be done in the NICU.

7. Surfactant administration

During fetal development, surfactant production starts at around 24–26 weeks' gestation with a continuous increase in production up to 36 weeks' gestation. At that time, the surfactant production is similar to that of adults. Term infants rarely require surfactant in the delivery room and surfactant should be given only after the infants have been admitted to the NICU. Using this approach will allow for a more gentle intubation with recued stress for the resuscitation team. Potential indications for surfactant administration include transient tachypnea of the newborn, meconium aspiration syndrome, respiratory distress syndrome, pulmonary hemorrhage, or presumed sepsis with secondary surfactant consumption.

8. Chest compressions

About 0.1% of term infants and up to 15% of preterm infants [76, 77] receive chest compression (CC) or epinephrine in the DR, which results in ~1 million newborn deaths annually worldwide. Infants who received epinephrine in the DR had a high incidence of mortality (41%) and short-term neurologic morbidity (57% hypoxic-ischemic encephalopathy and seizures) [78]. Furthermore, newborns receiving prolonged CC and epinephrine with no signs of life at 10 minutes following birth have up to 83% mortality, with 93% of survivors suffering moderate-to-severe disability [79]. Asphyxia could result from either failure of placental gas exchange before delivery (e.g., abruption and chorioamnionitis) or deficient pulmonary gas exchange immediately after birth (e.g., pulmonary hypertension) [80]. This condition of impaired gas exchange with simultaneous hypoxia and hypercapnia is leading to a mixed metabolic and respiratory acidosis [80]. Newborn infants are typically born with severe bradycardic or asystole. Current resuscitation guidelines recommend CC if the heart rate remains <60/min despite adequate PPV with 100% oxygen for 30 seconds; CC should be then performed at a rate of 90/min with 30 ventilations 3:1 C:V (compression:ventilation) ratio [4–6]. Rationales for using a 3:1 C:V ratio include (i) higher physiological heart rate (120–160/min) and breathing rates (40–60/min) in newborns compared to adults; (ii) profound bradycardia or cardiac arrest caused by hypoxia rather than primary cardiac compromise; therefore, providing ventilation is more likely to be beneficial in neonatal CPR compared to adult CPR [4–6].

However, the optimal C:V ratio that should be used during neonatal resuscitation to optimize coronary and cerebral perfusion while providing adequate ventilation of an asphyxiated newborn remains unknown [81]. Studies using newborn piglets with asphyxia-induced cardiac arrest demonstrated that combining CC with ventilations improves the return of spontaneous circulation (ROSC) and neurological outcome at 24 hours compared to ventilations or CC alone [16, 21]. Animal studies comparing various C:V ratios including 2:1 C:V, 4:1 C:V, 9:3 C:V, and 15:2 C:V to 3:1 C:V reported no difference in ROSC, survival or any other outcomes [82–84]. These studies suggest that during neonatal CPR, higher C:V ratios do not improve outcomes, and potentially a higher ventilation rate is needed. Similarly, *Schmölzer et al.* compared 3:1 C:V CPR with continuous CC with asynchronous ventilations (CCaV) using 90 CC and 30 non-synchronized inflations. The study reported similar time to ROSC (143 and 114 sec for 3:1 and CCaV, respectively), and survival (3/8 and 6/8, respectively) [85] suggesting no advantages of using CCaV compared to 3:1 C:V.

Most recently, a new technique providing CC during a sustained inflation (SI) (CC + SI) has been proposed, which significantly improved hemodynamics, minute ventilation, and time to ROSC compared to the 3:1 C:V ratio during resuscitation of asphyxiated newborn piglets [86]. While this first study used a CC rate of 120/min (in the CC + SI group) instead of the recommended 90/min, further studies using CC rates of 90/min in the same animal model have confirmed the initial findings [87–90]. Also a recent pilot trial in preterm infants <32 weeks' gestation showed similar results to the animal studies with a reduction in the mean (SD) time to ROSC with 31 (9) sec vs. 138 (72) sec in the CC + SI group and 3:1 C:V group (p = 0.011), respectively [91]. These data suggest that CC + SI has the potential to improve neonatal CPR, and a large randomized trial is currently ongoing to compare CC + SI with 3:1 C:V. Until these data are available, the 3:1 C:V ratio should be used during neonatal CPR.

9. Presence of parents during delivery room stabilization

There are no general rules about the presences of parents in delivery room during stabilization of their newborn. The approach chosen at any given facility will depend on (i) the local policy, (ii) geographical situation (e.g., separate stabilization room away from where the baby was delivered), and (iii) comfort of attending staff having parents in the room and observing the team. In addition, the increased use of smartphones and the urge of parents to photo document or video record, the resuscitation can add additional stress to the resuscitation team. In our institution, there is a geographical separation of the delivery suite and the stabilization room for high-risk deliveries. While the mother is unable to observe the resuscitation/stabilization, the father/partner would join the resuscitation team to be with their baby (father/partner is allowed to take photos, but not to video record) and would go back and forth between the stabilization room and the delivery suite to communicate with the mother. However, every hospital has to develop their own policy according to their needs to allow parents attendance during delivery and resuscitation.

10. Summary

Among the 15% of term babies who do not initiate spontaneous respirations after birth, 10% will require initial steps of stabilization: maintain normal temperature of the infant due to a dose-dependent increase in mortality for decreases of body temperature, position the infant in a "sniffing" position to open the airway, clear secretions with a bulb syringe or suction catheter if needed (if the airway appears obstructed or if PPV is required within 10–30 seconds of birth), dry the infant, and stimulate the infant (rubbing the back or the soles of the feet). Approximately 3% of term babies who do not initiate spontaneous respirations after birth will require PPV. Self-inflating bags, flow-inflating bags or T-piece devices may all be used for mask PPV, with currently limited evidence on the best device to be used to provide PPV in the DR. Among the interfaces, either face masks or nasal prongs could be used for PPV. Other interfaces that can be used are laryngeal mask and Guedel oropharyngeal airway. Lastly, approximately 2% of term babies who do not initiate spontaneous respirations after birth will be intubated and 0.1% will require CC and/or epinephrine to achieve this transition: current resuscitation guidelines recommend CC if the heart rate remains <60/min despite adequate PPV with 100% oxygen for 30 seconds; CC should be then performed at a rate of 90/min with a 3:1 C:V ratio. However, the optimal C:V ratio that should be used during neonatal resuscitation of an asphyxiated newborn remains unknown, with several ongoing studies assessing other techniques.

Author details

Francesca Viaroli[1] and Georg M. Schmölzer[1,2]*

*Address all correspondence to: georg.schmoelzer@me.com

1 Centre for the Studies of Asphyxia and Resuscitation, Royal Alexandra Hospital, Edmonton, Alberta, Canada

2 Department of Pediatrics, University of Alberta, Edmonton, Alberta, Canada

References

[1] Pas te A, Davis PG, Hooper SB, Morley CJ. From liquid to air: Breathing after birth. The Journal of Pediatrics. 2008;**152**:607-611

[2] Schmölzer GM, Pas te A, Davis PG, Morley CJ. Reducing lung injury during neonatal resuscitation of preterm infants. The Journal of Pediatrics. 2008;**153**:741-745

[3] Hooper SB, Siew ML, Kitchen M, Pas te A. Establishing functional residual capacity in the non-breathing infant. Seminars in Fetal & Neonatal Medicine. 2013;**18**:336-343

[4] Perlman JM, Wyllie JP, Kattwinkel J, Wyckoff MH, Aziz K, Guinsburg R, et al. Part 7: Neonatal resuscitation: 2015 international consensus on cardiopulmonary resuscitation and emergency cardiovascular care science with treatment recommendations. Circulation. 2015;**132**:S204-S241

[5] Wyckoff MH, Aziz K, Escobedo MB, Kattwinkel J, Perlman JM, Simon WM, et al. Part 13: Neonatal resuscitation: 2015 American Heart Association guidelines update for cardiopulmonary resuscitation and emergency cardiovascular care. American Heart Association. Circulation. 2015 Nov 3;**132**(18 Suppl 2):S543-S560

[6] Wyllie JP, Perlman JM, Kattwinkel J, Wyckoff MH, Aziz K, Guinsburg R, et al. Part 7: Neonatal resuscitation: 2015 international consensus on cardiopulmonary resuscitation and emergency cardiovascular care science with treatment recommendations. Resuscitation. 2015;**95**:e169-e201

[7] O'Donnell CPF, Kamlin COF, Davis PG, Morley CJ. Crying and breathing by extremely preterm infants immediately after birth. The Journal of Pediatrics. 2010;**156**:846-847

[8] Pas te A, Wong C, Kamlin COF, Dawson JA, Morley CJ, Davis PG. Breathing patterns in preterm and term infants immediately after birth. Pediatric Research. 2009;**65**:352-356

[9] Mullany LC. Neonatal hypothermia in low-resource settings. Seminars in Perinatology. 2010;**34**:426-433

[10] Mduma E, Ersdal H, Svensen E, Kidanto H, Auestad B, Perlman JM. Frequent brief on-site simulation training and reduction in 24-h neonatal mortality—An educational intervention study. Resuscitation. 2015;**93**:1-7

[11] Ersdal HL, Mduma E, Svensen E, Perlman JM. Early initiation of basic resuscitation interventions including face mask ventilation may reduce birth asphyxia related mortality in low-income countries. Resuscitation. 2012;**83**:869-873

[12] Dekker J, Martherus T, Cramer SJE, van Zanten HA, Hooper SB, Pas te A. Tactile stimulation to stimulate spontaneous breathing during stabilization of preterm infants at birth: A retrospective analysis. Frontiers in Pediatrics. 2017;**5**:457-456

[13] Dekker J, Hooper SB, Martherus T, Cramer SJE, van Geloven N, Pas te A. Repetitive versus standard tactile stimulation of preterm infants at birth – A randomized controlled trial. Resuscitation. 2018;**127**:37-43

[14] East CE, Colditz PB, Begg LM, Brennecke SP. Update on intrapartum fetal pulse oximetry. The Australian & New Zealand Journal of Obstetrics & Gynaecology. 2002;**42**:119-124

[15] Dawson JA, Kamlin COF, Vento M, Wong C, Cole TJ, Donath S, et al. Defining the reference range for oxygen saturation for infants after birth. Pediatrics. 2010;**125**:e1340-e1347

[16] Kattwinkel J, Perlman JM, Aziz K, Colby C, Fairchild K, Gallagher J, et al. Part 15: Neonatal resuscitation: 2010 American Heart Association guidelines for cardiopulmonary resuscitation and emergency cardiovascular care. Circulation. 2010;**122**:S909-S919

[17] Dawson JA, Ekström A, Frisk C, Thio M, Roehr C-C, Kamlin COF, et al. Assessing the tongue colour of newly born infants may help to predict the need for supplemental oxygen in the delivery room. Acta Paediatrica. 2015 Apr;**104**(4):356-359

[18] O'Donnell CPF, Kamlin COF, Davis PG, Carlin JB, Morley CJ. Clinical assessment of infant colour at delivery. Archives of Disease in Childhood. Fetal and Neonatal. 2007;**92**:F465-F467

[19] O'Donnell CPF, Kamlin COF, Davis PG, Carlin JB, Morley CJ. Interobserver variability of the 5-minute Apgar score. The Journal of Pediatrics. 2006;**149**:486-489

[20] Tan A, Schulze A, O'Donnell CPF, Davis PG. Air versus oxygen for resuscitation of infants at birth. Cochrane Database of Systematic Reviews. 2005 Apr;**18**(2):CD002273

[21] Davis PG, Tan A, O'Donnell CPF, Schulze A. Resuscitation of newborn infants with 100% oxygen or air: A systematic review and meta-analysis. The Lancet. 2004;**364**:1329-1333

[22] Aziz K, Chadwick M, Baker M, Andrews W. Ante- and intra-partum factors that predict increased need for neonatal resuscitation. Resuscitation. 2008;**79**:444-452

[23] Finer N, Rich W, Wang CL, Leone TA. Airway obstruction during mask ventilation of very low birth weight infants during neonatal resuscitation. Pediatrics. 2009;**123**:865-869

[24] Schmölzer GM, Dawson JA, Kamlin COF, O'Donnell CPF, Morley CJ, Davis PG. Airway obstruction and gas leak during mask ventilation of preterm infants in the delivery room. Archives of Disease in Childhood. Fetal and Neonatal. 2011;**96**:F254-F257

[25] Cheung D, Mian QN, Cheung P-Y, Reilly MOA, Aziz K, van Os S, et al. Mask ventilation with two different face masks in the delivery room for preterm infants: A randomized controlled trial. Journal of Perinatology. 2015;**35**:1-5

[26] Schmölzer GM, Kamlin COF, O'Donnell CPF, Dawson JA, Morley CJ, Davis PG. Assessment of tidal volume and gas leak during mask ventilation of preterm infants in the delivery room. Archives of Disease in Childhood. Fetal and Neonatal. 2010;**95**:F393-F397

[27] Poulton DA, Schmölzer GM, Morley CJ, Davis PG. Assessment of chest rise during mask ventilation of preterm infants in the delivery room. Resuscitation. 2011;**82**:175-179

[28] Kaufman J, Schmölzer GM, Kamlin COF, Davis PG. Mask ventilation of preterm infants in the delivery room. Archives of Disease in Childhood. Fetal and Neonatal. 2013;**98**:F405-F410

[29] Schilleman K, van der Pot CJM, Hooper SB, Lopriore E, Walther FJ, Pas te A. Evaluating manual inflations and breathing during mask ventilation in preterm infants at birth. The Journal of Pediatrics. 2013;**162**:457-463

[30] Chua C, Schmölzer GM, Davis PG. Airway manoeuvres to achieve upper airway patency during mask ventilation in newborn infants – An historical perspective. Resuscitation. 2012;**83**:411-416

[31] Hawkes CP, Ryan CA, Dempsey EM. Comparison of the T-piece resuscitator with other neonatal manual ventilation devices: A qualitative review. Resuscitation. 2012;**83**:797-802

[32] Morley CJ, Dawson JA, Stewart M, Hussain F, Davis PG. The effect of a PEEP valve on a Laerdal neonatal self-inflating resuscitation bag. Journal of Paediatrics and Child Health. 2010;**46**:51-56

[33] Szyld E, Aguilar AM, Musante GA, Vain NE, Prudent L, Fabres J, et al. Comparison of devices for newborn ventilation in the delivery room. The Journal of Pediatrics. 2014;**165**: 234-239.e3

[34] Dawson JA, Schmölzer GM, Kamlin COF, Pas te A, O'Donnell CPF, Donath S, et al. Oxygenation with T-piece versus self-inflating bag for ventilation of extremely preterm infants at birth: A randomized controlled trial. The Journal of Pediatrics. 2011;**158**:912-918.e1-2

[35] Bennett S, Finer N, Rich W, Vaucher Y. A comparison of three neonatal resuscitation devices. Resuscitation. 2005;**67**:113-118

[36] Finer NN, Barrington KJ, Al-Fadley F, Peters KL. Limitations of self-inflating resuscitators. Pediatrics. 1986 Mar;**77**(3):417-420. Available from: http://pediatrics.aappublications.org/content/77/3/417.short

[37] Wyllie JP, Oddie S, Scally A. Use of self-inflating bags for neonatal resuscitation. Resuscitation. 2005;**67**:109-112

[38] Dawson JA, Gerber A, Kamlin COF, Davis PG, Morley CJ. Providing PEEP during neonatal resuscitation: Which device is best? Journal of Paediatrics and Child Health. 2011;**47**:698-703

[39] Klingenberg C, Dawson JA, Gerber A, Kamlin COF, Davis PG, Morley CJ. Sustained inflations: Comparing three neonatal resuscitation devices. Neonatology. 2011;**100**:78-84

[40] Wyllie JP, Nolan JP, Soar J, Zideman D, Biarent D, Bossaert LL, et al. European resuscitation council guidelines for resuscitation 2010 section 1. Executive summary. Resuscitation. 2010;**81**:1219-1276

[41] Field D, Milner AD, Hopkin IE. Efficiency of manual resuscitators at birth. Archives of Disease in Childhood. 1986;**61**:300-302

[42] Hooper SB, Fouras A, Siew ML, Wallace MJ, Kitchen M, Pas te A, et al. Expired CO2 levels indicate degree of lung aeration at birth. PLoS One. 2013;**8**:e70895

[43] Schmölzer GM, Hooper SB, Wong C, Kamlin COF, Davis PG. Exhaled carbon dioxide in healthy term infants immediately after birth. The Journal of Pediatrics. 2015;**166**:844-9.e1-3

[44] Schmölzer GM, Morley CJ, Wong C, Dawson JA, Kamlin COF, Donath S, et al. Respiratory function monitor guidance of mask ventilation in the delivery room: A feasibility study. The Journal of Pediatrics. 2012;**160**:377-381.e2

[45] McCarthy LK, O'Donnell CPF, Twomey AR, Molloy EJ, Murphy JFA. A randomized trial of nasal prong or face mask for respiratory support for preterm newborns. Pediatrics. 2013;**132**:e389-e395

[46] Kamlin COF, Schilleman K, Dawson JA, Lopriore E, Donath S, Schmölzer GM, et al. Mask versus nasal tube for stabilization of preterm infants at birth: A randomized controlled trial. Pediatrics. 2013;**132**:e381-e388

[47] Wood FE, Morley CJ, Dawson JA, Davis PG. A respiratory function monitor improves mask ventilation. Archives of Disease in Childhood. Fetal and Neonatal. 2008;**93**:F380-F381

[48] Wood FE, Dawson JA, Morley CJ, Kamlin COF, Owen LS, Donath S, et al. Assessing the effectiveness of two round neonatal resuscitation masks: Study 1. Archives of Disease in Childhood. Fetal and Neonatal. 2008;**93**:F235-F237

[49] Wood FE, Morley CJ. Face mask ventilation–the dos and don'ts. Seminars in Fetal & Neonatal Medicine. 2013;**18**:344-351

[50] Schmölzer GM, Olischar M, Raith W, Resch B, Reiterer F, Müller W. Delivery room resuscitation. Monatsschrift für Kinderheilkunde. 2010;**158**:471-476

[51] Leone TA, Rich W, Finer N. A survey of delivery room resuscitation practices in the United States. Pediatrics. 2006;**117**:e164-e175

[52] Vento M, Iriondo M, Thio M, Burón E, Salguero E, Aguayo J, et al. A survey of neonatal resuscitation in Spain: Gaps between guidelines and practice. Acta Paediatrica. 2009;**98**: 786-791

[53] O'Shea JE, Thio M, Owen LS, Wong C, Dawson JA, Davis PG. Measurements from preterm infants to guide face mask size. Archives of Disease in Childhood. Fetal and Neonatal. 2016;**101**:F294-F298

[54] Brain AI. The laryngeal mask–a new concept in airway management. British Journal of Anaesthesia. 1983 Aug;**55**(8):801-805

[55] Barata I. The laryngeal mask airway: Prehospital and emergency department use. Emergency Medicine Clinics of North America. 2008 Nov;**26**(4):1069-1083

[56] Joshi GP, Joshi GP, Inagaki Y, White PF, Taylor-Kennedy L. Use of the laryngeal mask airway as an alternative to the tracheal tube during ambulatory anesthesia. Anesthesia and Analgesia. 1997 Sep;**85**(3):573-577

[57] Schmölzer GM, Agarwal M, Kamlin COF, Davis PG. Supraglottic airway devices during neonatal resuscitation: An historical perspective, systematic review and meta-analysis of available clinical trials. Resuscitation. 2013;**84**:722-730

[58] Bansal SC, Caoci S, Dempsey EM, Trevisanuto D, Roehr C-C. The laryngeal mask airway and its use in neonatal resuscitation: A critical review of where we are in 2017/2018. Neonatology. 2018;**113**(2):152-161. DOI: 10.1159/000481979

[59] Trevisanuto D, Verghese C, Doglioni N, Ferrarese P, Zanardo V. Laryngeal mask airway for the interhospital transport of neonates. Pediatrics. 2005 Jan;**115**(1):e109-11. Epub 2004 Dec 15

[60] Brimacombe JR, De Maio B. Emergency use of the laryngeal mask airway during helicopter transfer of a neonate. Journal of Clinical Anesthesia. 1995;**7**:689-690

[61] Fraser J, Hill C, McDonald D, Jones C, Petros A. The use of the laryngeal mask airway for inter-hospital transport of infants with type 3 laryngotracheo-oesophageal clefts. Intensive Care Medicine. 1999 Jul;**25**(7):714-716

[62] Bucx MJL, Grolman W, Kruisinga FH, Lindeboom JAH, Van Kempen AAMW. The prolonged use of the laryngeal mask airway in a neonate with airway obstruction and Treacher Collins syndrome. Pediatric Anesthesia. 2003;**13**:530-533

[63] Fernández-Jurado M, Fernández-Baena M. Use of laryngeal mask airway for prolonged ventilatory support in a preterm newborn. Paediatric Anaesthesia 2002 May;**12**(4):369-370

[64] Udaeta ME, Weiner GM. Alternative ventilation strategies: Laryngeal masks. Clinics in Perinatology. 2006;**33**:99-110

[65] Micaglio M, Zanardo V, Ori C, Parotto M, Doglioni N, Trevisanuto D. ProSeal LMA for surfactant administration. Pediatric Anesthesia. 2007;**18**:91-92

[66] Trevisanuto D, Grazzina N, Ferrarese P, Micaglio M, Verghese C, Zanardo V. Laryngeal mask airway used as a delivery conduit for the Administration of Surfactant to preterm infants with respiratory distress syndrome. Biology of the Neonate. 2005;**87**:217-220

[67] Pinheiro JM, Santana-Rivas Q, Pezzano C. Randomized trial of laryngeal mask airway versus endotracheal intubation for surfactant delivery. Journal of Perinatology. 2016 Mar; **36**(3):196-201. DOI: 10.1038/jp.2015.177. Epub 2015 Dec 3

[68] Lin H-J, Chen K-T, Liao C-K, Foo N-P, Lin C-C, Guo H-R. Epinephrine administration via a laryngeal mask airway: What is the optimal dose? Signa Vitae. 2010;**5**:25-28

[69] Chen K-T, Lin H-J, Guo H-R, Lin M-T, Lin C-C. Feasibility study of epinephrine administration via laryngeal mask airway using a porcine model. Resuscitation. 2006;**69**:503-507

[70] Marsh AM, Nunn JF, Taylor SJ, Charlesworth CH. Airway obstruction associated with the use of the Guedel airway. British Journal of Anaesthesia. 1991 Nov;**67**(5):517-523

[71] Wyllie JP, Richmond S. European resuscitation council guidelines for resuscitation 2010. Resuscitation. 2010;**81**:1389-1399

[72] Fortin G, Oulton J. Evaluation of methods of resuscitation. Canadian Anaesthetists' Society Journal. 1955 October;**2**(4):354-361

[73] Donald I. Resuscitation of the newborn. Postgraduate Medical Journal. 1953 May;**29**(331): 247-253

[74] Vasey PM. Asphyxia Neonatorum. The Journal of the College of General Practitioners. 1963;**6**:373-394

[75] O'Donnell CPF, Davis PG, Morley CJ. Use of supplementary equipment for resuscitation of newborn infants at tertiary perinatal centres in Australia and New Zealand. Acta Paediatrica. 2005

[76] Wyckoff MH, Perlman JM. Cardiopulmonary resuscitation in very low birth weight infants. Pediatrics. 2000;**106**:618-620

[77] Soraisham AS, Lodha AK, Singhal N, Aziz K, Yang J, Lee SK, et al. Neonatal outcomes following extensive cardiopulmonary resuscitation in the delivery room for infants born at less than 33 weeks gestational age. Resuscitation. 2014;**85**:238-243

[78] Barber CA, Wyckoff MH. Use and efficacy of endotracheal versus intravenous epinephrine during neonatal cardiopulmonary resuscitation in the delivery room. Pediatrics. 2006; **118**:1028-1034

[79] Harrington DJ, Redman CW, Moulden M, Greenwood CE. The long-term outcome in surviving infants with Apgar zero at 10 minutes: A systematic review of the literature and hospital-based cohort. American Journal of Obstetrics and Gynecology. 2007;**196**:463. e1-463.e5

[80] Wyckoff MH. Chest compressions for bradycardia or asystole in neonates. Clinics in Perinatology. 2012;**39**:833-842

[81] Wyckoff MH, Berg RA. Optimizing chest compressions during delivery-room resuscitation. Seminars in Fetal & Neonatal Medicine. 2008;**13**:410-415

[82] Solevåg AL, Dannevig I, Wyckoff MH, Saugstad OD, Nakstad B. Extended series of cardiac compressions during CPR in a swine model of perinatal asphyxia. Resuscitation. 2010;**81**:1571-1576

[83] Solevåg AL, Dannevig I, Wyckoff MH, Saugstad OD, Nakstad B. Return of spontaneous circulation with a compression: Ventilation ratio of 15:2 versus 3:1 in newborn pigs with cardiac arrest due to asphyxia. Archives of Disease in Childhood. Fetal and Neonatal. 2011;**96**:F417-F421

[84] Pasquin MP, Cheung PY, Patel S, Lu M, Lee TF, Wagner M, O'Reilly M, Schmölzer GM. Comparison of different compression to ventilation ratios (2:1, 3:1, and 4:1) during cardiopulmonary resuscitation in a porcine model of neonatal asphyxia. Neonatology. 2018; **114**(1):37-45

[85] Schmölzer GM, O'Reilly M, LaBossiere J, Lee T-F, Cowan S, Nicoll J, et al. 3:1 compression to ventilation ratio versus continuous chest compression with asynchronous ventilation in a porcine model of neonatal resuscitation. Resuscitation. 2014;**85**:270-275

[86] Schmölzer GM, O'Reilly M, LaBossiere J, Lee T-F, Cowan S, Qin S, et al. Cardiopulmonary resuscitation with chest compressions during sustained inflations: A new technique of neonatal resuscitation that improves recovery and survival in a neonatal porcine model. Circulation. 2013;**128**:2495-2503

[87] Li ES-S, Cheung P-Y, O'Reilly M, Aziz K, Schmölzer GM. Rescuer fatigue during simulated neonatal cardiopulmonary resuscitation. Journal of Perinatology. 2015;**35**:142-145

[88] Solevåg AL, Cheung P-Y, Li ES-S, Aziz K, O'Reilly M, Fu B, et al. Quantifying force application to a newborn manikin during simulated cardiopulmonary resuscitation. Journal of Maternal-Fetal and Neonatal Medicine. 2016;**29**:1770-1772

[89] Li ES-S, Cheung P-Y, Lee T-F, Lu M, O'Reilly M, Schmölzer GM. Return of spontaneous circulation is not affected by different chest compression rates superimposed with sustained inflations during cardiopulmonary resuscitation in newborn piglets. PLoS One. 2016;**11**:e0157249-e0157214

[90] Li ES-S, Görens I, Cheung P-Y, Lee T-F, Lu M, O'Reilly M, et al. Chest compressions during sustained inflations improve recovery when compared to a 3:1 compression:Ventilation ratio during cardiopulmonary resuscitation in a neonatal porcine model of asphyxia. Neonatology. 2017;**112**:337-346

[91] Schmölzer GM, O'Reilly M, Fray C, van Os S, Cheung P-Y. Chest compression during sustained inflation versus 3:1 chest compression: Ventilation ratio during neonatal cardiopulmonary resuscitation: A randomised feasibility trial. Archives of Disease in Childhood. Fetal and Neonatal. 2017

Chapter 4

Ultrasound-Guided Vascular Access during Cardiopulmonary Resuscitation

Anton Kasatkin, Aleksandr Urakov and Anna Nigmatullina

Additional information is available at the end of the chapter

http://dx.doi.org/10.5772/intechopen.79400

Abstract

The chapter considers the possibilities for using ultrasound to increase the efficiency and safety of the intravascular access in patients during cardiac arrest, cardiopulmonary resuscitation, and advanced life support. It provides the grounds for the real-time use of ultrasound for ensuring satisfactory central vascular access; the main principles of this methodology and current recommendations are described as well. In addition, the article presents special aspects of visualization of ultrasound vessels in cardiopulmonary resuscitation, as well as puncture and catheterization techniques. It is crucial that resuscitators, who are often at the forefront of patient resuscitation, understand how to properly use this potentially life-saving procedure.

Keywords: cardiopulmonary resuscitation, advanced life support, ultrasound, vascular access, vascular visualization

1. Introduction

Providing satisfactory vascular access is still a critical part of resuscitation. Timely administration of drugs through intravenous access can improve the survival rate of patients after circulatory arrest. The time passed from the arrest to drug administration is an independent predictor of return to the spontaneous circulation [1]. In this regard, it is difficult to overestimate the importance of providing satisfactory vascular access for the patient with circulatory arrest. It is important to remember that the benefits of early vascular access must be considered together with the importance of uninterrupted cardiopulmonary resuscitation (CPR) [2]. When choosing vascular access, it is a common practice firstly to focus on visualization and palpation of the

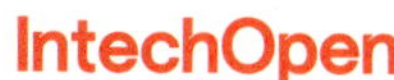

subcutaneous veins in the accessible parts of the body, as well as on the anatomical landmark (landmark technique). Subcutaneous veins in the extremities and the external jugular veins completely satisfy these requirements. The insertion of the catheter into visualized subcutaneous vein is considered to be quick and safe. It should be remembered that visualization and palpation of the subcutaneous veins can be difficult in patients in critical condition (bleeding, hypovolemic shock, burns of limbs, or hypothermia). In this case, infrared thermography [3] and near-infrared vein visualization [4] can be applied. If the catheterization of the subcutaneous veins is difficult or impossible, then intraosseous access (IO) is recommended by current clinical guidelines [5]. Nowadays, IO route is proved to be quite effective in adults and children with out-of-hospital cardiac arrest [6]. It is assumed that insertion of a central venous catheter requires the interruption of CPR and can be technically challenging and associated with complications. However, the introduction of real-time ultrasound-guided central venous catheter (CVC) insertion into clinical practice significantly increased its safety, accuracy, and effectiveness compared to the conventional landmark technique [7, 8]. It is known that central venous access is required for administering drug solutions, monitoring venous pressure, and for performing extracorporeal oxygenation and detoxification, which cannot be achieved by other types of access. In addition, ultrasound-guided catheterization of the internal jugular (IJV) and femoral veins (FV) may not require the cessation of chest compression and placing a patient in a forced position (head-down tilt positions) during CPR. It is critical that resuscitators, who are often at the forefront of patient resuscitation, understand how to properly use this potentially life-saving procedure.

2. History

The use of ultrasound imaging support for IJV location was first described in 1978 [9]. The use of ultrasound for real-time CVC insertion was reported in 1984. Legler and Nugent [10] showed that Doppler localization of the IJV facilitates central venous cannulation. Later, the results of studies showing the advantage of using ultrasound for catheterization of subclavian (SV) and FV were published [11]. The first results of studies on the use of ultrasound for catheterization of the central vein during CPR were published in 1997. Hilty et al. [12] showed that real-time ultrasound-guided FV catheterization was faster and produced a lower rate of inadvertent arterial catheterization and a higher rate of success during CPR than the standard landmark-oriented approach. Benassi et al. [13] showed the benefits of the real-time ultrasound cannulation of the femoral vessels for establishing venoarterial extracorporeal membrane oxygenation in acute cardiopulmonary failure.

3. Principles of vessel visualization using ultrasound

Two-dimensional (2D) gray-scale imaging (**Figure 1**), color (**Figure 2**), and spectral Doppler (**Figure 3**) ultrasonography are used for ultrasonic visualization of vascular structures, surrounding tissues, and anatomical formations [14]. The best resolution of surface structures in the immediate vicinity of the skin surface is provided by high-frequency (>7 MHz) linear ultrasonic sensors. The operator must have an idea of the probe orientation, the image on

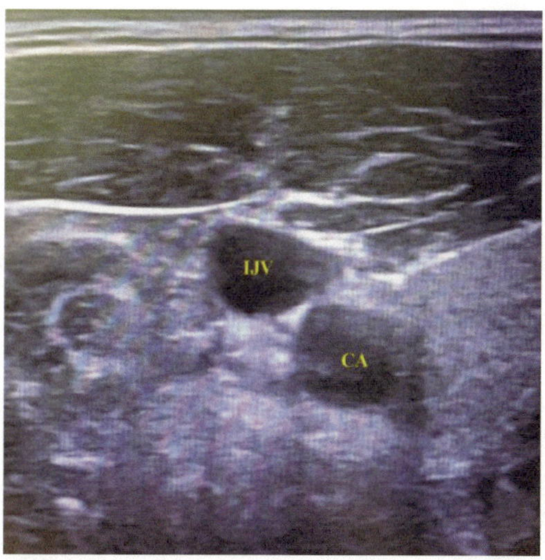

Figure 1. Ultrasound 2D image of the right internal jugular vein (IJV) and carotid artery (CA).

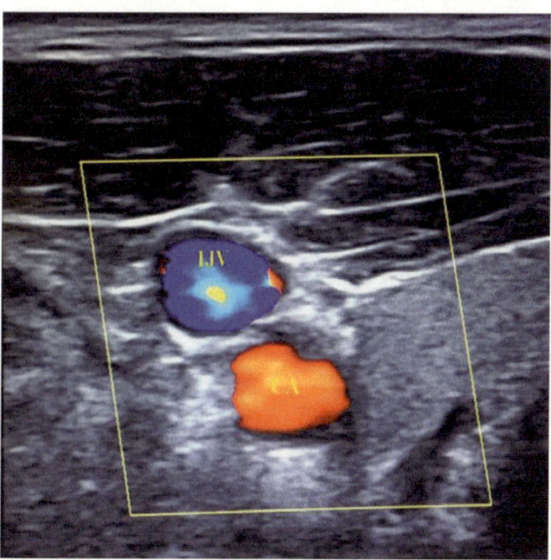

Figure 2. Ultrasound color Doppler imaging of the right internal jugular vein (IJV) and carotid artery (CA).

the display, the physics of ultrasound, the mechanism of image generation, and the artifacts, and be able to interpret 2D images of the vessel lumen and surrounding structures. A two-dimensional image of a blood vessel is usually displayed either along the long axis (**Figure 4**), the short axis (**Figure 5**) or the oblique short axis (**Figure 6**).

3.1. Ultrasonic visualization of blood vessels in people with spontaneous circulation

The basic differences between a vein and an artery in an ultrasound 2D image are the irregular form of the vein (the artery is generally round) and the wall thickness (the arterial walls are

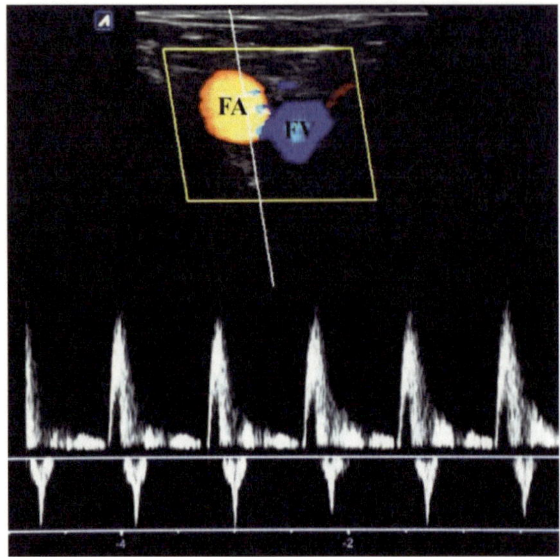

Figure 3. Ultrasound color Doppler and spectral Doppler imaging of the right femoral artery (FA) and femoral vein (FV).

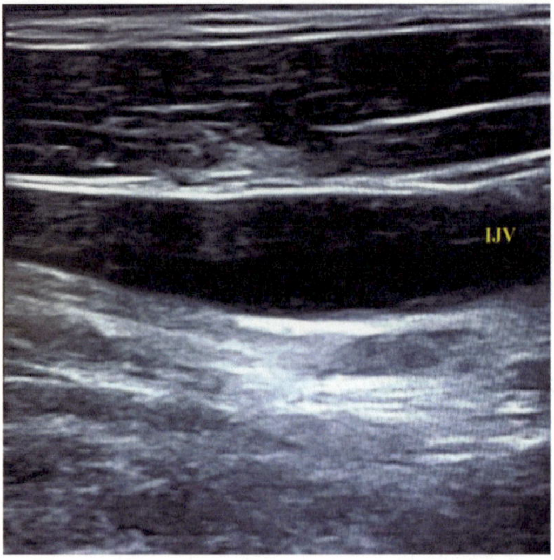

Figure 4. A two-dimensional image of the right internal jugular vein (IJV) along the long axis view.

thicker), but the major difference is vein compressibility under a slight external surface pressure (**Figures 7** and **8**). The lack of vein compressibility may indicate the presence of a thrombus. Using Doppler also helps to distinguish a vein from an artery. Respiratory-based vein excursion may also allow us to distinguish it from the artery [15]. Respiratory-based vein excursion is a change in its diameter based on the respiration phase. It is known that, in contrast to the arteries, the IJV, SV, and FV diameter decreases during inhalation and increases during exhalation [16]. In patients with hypovolemia, the IJV may completely collapse during inhalation

http://dx.doi.org/10.5772/intechopen.79400

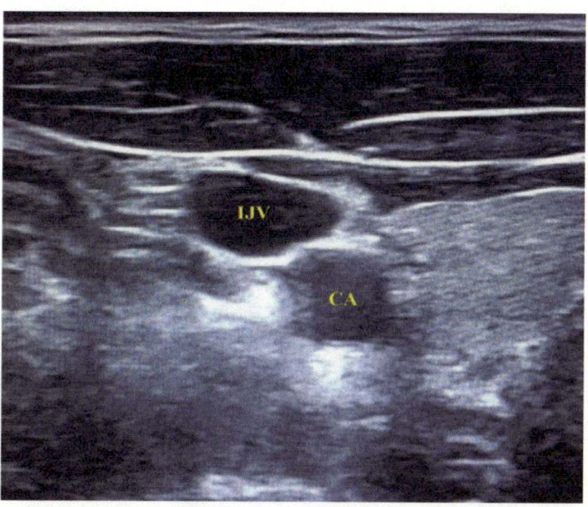

Figure 5. A two-dimensional image of the right internal jugular vein (IJV) and carotid artery (CA) along the short axis view.

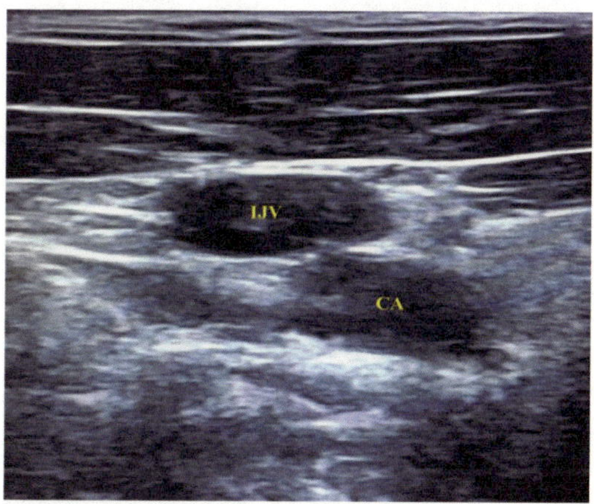

Figure 6. A two-dimensional image of the right internal jugular vein (IJV) and carotid artery (CA) along the oblique short view.

(**Figure 9**). It must be remembered that the color does not determine the nature of the blood flow (venous or arterial), but depends on the flow direction (from the probe or to the probe). By default, the device marks the blood flow directed toward the probe as red, and the blood flowing away from the probe is marked as blue. The change in the inclination of the probe can lead to the change in the vessel color on the screen of the ultrasonic device.

3.2. Special aspects of ultrasound imaging of vessels during cardiac arrest and CPR

During circulatory arrest, the blood pressure on the walls of arteries decreases; they lose elasticity and are compressed together with veins when external surface pressure is applied by the ultrasonic probe. In this regard, compressibility during cardiac arrest is characteristic of both the vein and the artery. When performing chest compression, the blood pressure on the

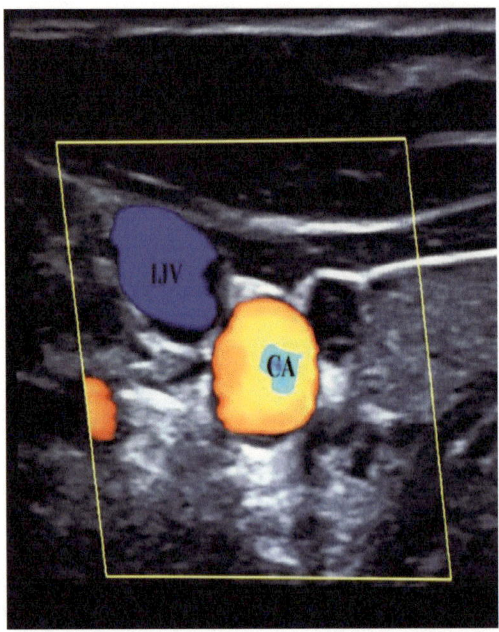

Figure 7. Ultrasound color Doppler imaging of the right internal jugular vein (IJV) and carotid artery (CA) before external surface pressure.

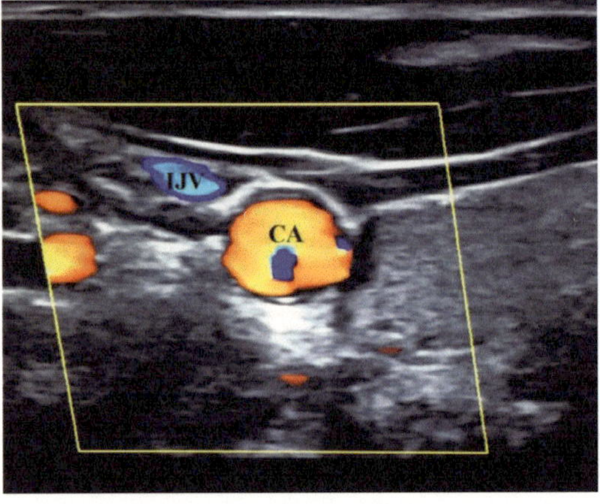

Figure 8. Ultrasound color Doppler imaging of the right internal jugular vein (IJV) and carotid artery (CA) after external surface pressure.

walls in the arteries increases. An increase in blood pressure (more than 60 mmHg) leads to an increase in the elasticity of the arteries walls, which again makes them noncompressible when pressed [17]. During CPR rhythmic change in diameter is typical for both veins and arteries due to compression and decompression of the chest with a frequency of 100–120 per minute (diameter of the CA may change by 30–40% and IJV by 50–60%). Using a Doppler is a reliable way to distinguish the artery from the vein by the flow direction.

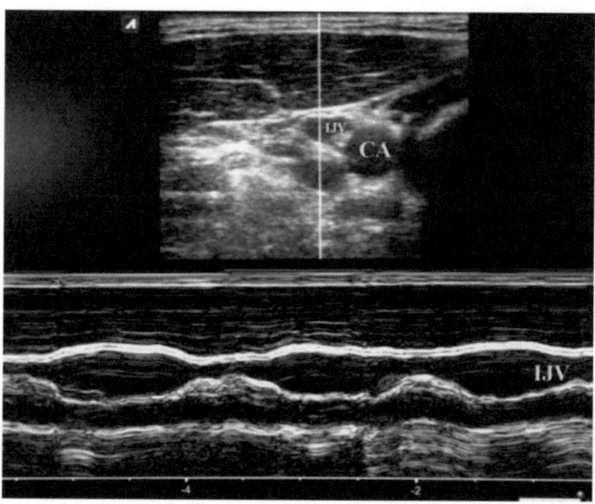

Figure 9. Measuring right internal jugular vein (IJV) diameter in healthy volunteer using M-mode ultrasonography.

The ratio of the sizes (diameters) of IJV, SV, and FV veins in patients with cardiac arrest may vary. If the cause of cardiac arrest is hypovolemia (blood loss), then the ratio of the veins diameter will be as follows: IJV < SV > FV. If the cause of cardiac arrest was thromboembolism, acute myocardial infarction or tamponade, the ratio of the veins diameter will be different: FV < SV > IJV.

4. IJV anatomy, access, and catheterization technique

IJV emerges from the outer jugular opening at the base of the skull posterior to the internal carotid artery (CA), then proceeds caudally, and shifts, taking anterolateral position in regards to CA. Denys and Uretsky [18] showed that the IJ was located anterolateral in regards to CA in 92% (**Figure 7**), >1 cm lateral to the carotid in 1%, medial to the carotid in 2%, and outside of the path predicted by landmarks in 5.5% of patients. Preliminary ultrasound evaluation of the vein patency, size, location, and possible anomalies is mandatory, it ensures avoiding futile attempts as in patients whose IJV is absent or thrombosed or who have congenital anomalies. Surrounding structures (subcutaneous tissue, carotid artery, thyroid, and lymph nodes) must also be analyzed. The properly trained clinicians use real-time ultrasound during IJV cannulation whenever possible to improve cannulation success and reduce the incidence of complications associated with the insertion of large bore catheters. Before the procedure, a patient should be placed in position on his back. The head can be turned to the contralateral side from 0 to 40°. The head-down tilt position should be used, when possible, for increasing the vein size, eliminating the vein respiratory excursion, reducing the risk of air embolism during IJV cannulation, and consequently improving the success of CVC insertion. For more than 65% of patients requiring CVC, the 10° head-down tilt position is sufficient to increase the size of IJV. In certain clinical situations, the head-down tilt position may not be applied.

4.1. Approach to vein puncture

Currently, three types of approach for real-time ultrasound-guided IJV catheterization are described: central (classical), lateral, and lateral oblique.

For classical IJV approach, one can use short or long axis vein visualization and in-plane (when included in the plane of the ultrasound beam) or out-of-plane (only a very limited part of the needle can be visualized by the ultrasound beam) needle visualization [14]. The long axis view of the IJV can be obtained by positioning the ultrasound probe in longitudinal orientation on the patient's neck. This view shows the course of the IJV, and with this probe positioning, the needle is inserted in-plane at the level of the cranial edge of the ultrasound probe; this allows the operator to visualize the entire length of the needle through the soft tissue and into the IJV [19]. With this type of technique, the information of the carotid artery, lymph nodes, and thyroid may be lost. In addition, the IJV access will be at least 3 cm cranial from the upper margin of the clavicle, for the limitation imposed by the ultrasound probe length. This fact makes it difficult to apply this kind of approach in patients with a short neck. The short axis view of the vein can be obtained by positioning the ultrasound probe in a transverse orientation (90° rotation from the long axis) on the patient's neck (the ultrasound probe is perpendicular to the course of the IJV). This view allows the visualization of the carotid artery, lymph nodes, and thyroid. With this position of the ultrasound probe, the needle is usually inserted vertically (vertical out-of-plane technique) above the middle part of the ultrasound probe in a position 1–1.5 cm cranial from the upper margin of the clavicle. This allows the operator to simultaneously visualize the IJV and all surrounding structures and ensures a caudal vein access [20]. With this type of technique, the operator has a very limited view of the needle (**Figure 10**).

The lateral short axis in-plane technique is a combination of the advantages of both previously mentioned conventional techniques, but without their limitations [21]. The ultrasound probe is positioned in a transverse orientation (short axis), with a good view of the IJV and its surrounding structures. The needle is inserted at the level of the lateral edge of the ultrasound probe [22]. This guarantees the visualization of the entire length of the needle during vein access (**Figure 11**).

This allows the operator to avoid iatrogenic puncture complications, such as arterial puncture and pneumothorax. The ultrasound-guided lateral short axis in-plane technique for percutaneous IJV cannulation can be successfully applied in patients without hypovolemia. Using this method for patients with hypovolemia and veins with a small diameter (less than 7 mm) may result in vein perforation [23].

The real-time ultrasound-guided lateral oblique short axis in-plane technique may be successfully applied in patients with hypovolemia and a small IJV size. The lateral oblique short axis view of the vein can be obtained by positioning the ultrasound probe rotated in 10–50° from the short axis. This method can be applied as follows: set the sensor so that the vein image in the transverse axis is located in the middle of the screen of the ultrasound scanner and measure the maximum distance between the lateral and medial walls at the time of inspiration of the patient. If this distance is less than 7 mm, the sensor is rotated by moving

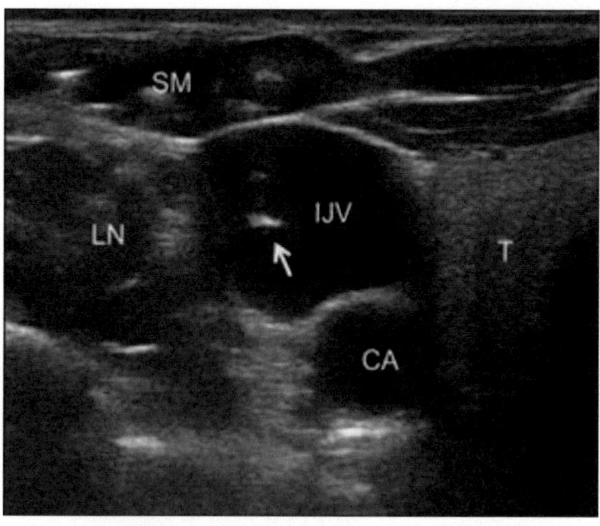

Figure 10. Short axis vertical out-of-plane technique ultrasound image of the right neck area showing the internal jugular vein (IJV), carotid artery (CA), lymph nodes (LN), sternocleidomastoid muscle (SM), and the thyroid (T). The needle is visible in a limited fashion into the internal jugular vein as a bright dot (arrow). From J Vasc Access [22].

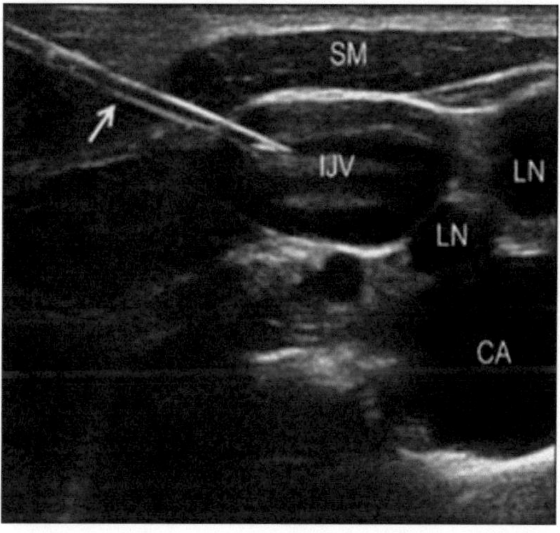

Figure 11. Short axis, lateral in-plane technique ultrasound image of the right neck area showing the internal jugular vein (IJV), carotid artery (CA), lymph nodes (LN), and the sternocleidomastoid muscle (SM). The needle is visible in its entire length with the full tip into the internal jugular vein (arrow). From J Vasc Access [22].

its lateral part upwards and the medial part downwards, and the rotation of the sensor is stopped when the distance between the walls of the vein is more than 7 mm. Fix the sensor in this position. Puncture needle is then inserted, and the vein is punctured in the sensor plane. [24]. This maneuver allows us to increase the size of the vein compared to the size in short axis (**Figure 12**).

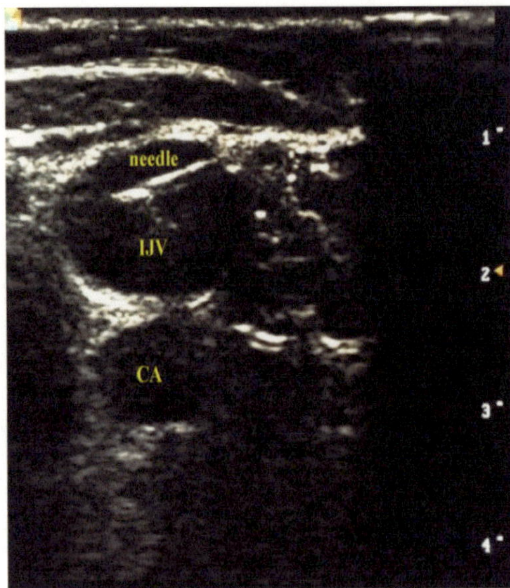

Figure 12. Lateral oblique short axis in-plane technique ultrasound image of the internal jugular vein (IJV), carotid artery (CA), and needle is visible in its entire length with the full tip into the internal jugular vein.

5. FV and FA anatomy, access, and catheterization techniques

Common femoral vein and common femoral artery (FA) lie within the femoral triangle formed by the inguinal ligament, the long adductor muscle, and the sartorius muscle. An important landmark for determining the location of the femoral vein in patients with spontaneous circulation is the femoral artery pulsation, since the vein is usually located medial to the artery in the vascular lacuna of the femoral triangle. This vascular interposition is constant only under the inguinal ligament (**Figure 13**). Change in the relative location of the vessels occurs in the caudal direction. In particular, the FA may overlap the femoral vein at a level of 1 cm below the inguinal ligament. In this regard, ultrasound imaging will accurately localize the FV and differentiate it from the femoral artery (**Figure 14**).

During CPR, it is possible to reliably distinguish the artery from the vein during the chest compression in the direction of the flow with the help of the Doppler. The advantages of choosing a femoral vein are the possibility to perform its catheterization without disrupting the CPR, lack of control devices in this area, and the ability for the resuscitator to access the patient's chest and airways. In addition, this access prevents pneumo- and hemothorax. Well-known complications of catheterization are vascular damage, bleeding, and arteriovenous fistulas.

Before the catheterization, the patient should be placed on his back, with his thigh slightly retracted, and rotated outwards. This technique allows us to increase the accessibility of the common femoral vein in 70–80% of adults [25]. It is possible to increase the cross-sectional

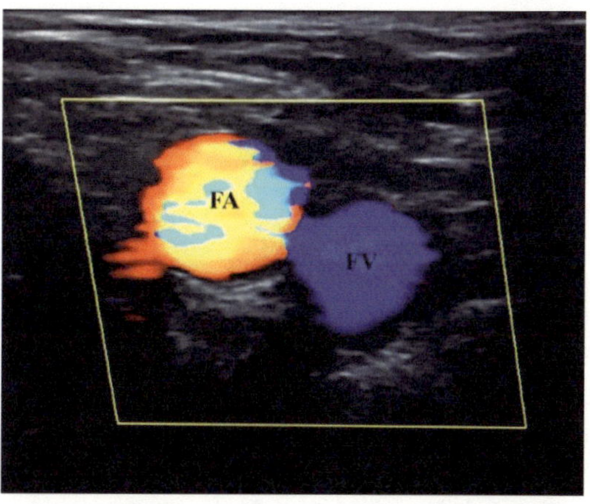

Figure 13. Ultrasound color Doppler imaging of the right femoral artery (FA) and femoral vein (FV). The US probe is installed under the inguinal ligament.

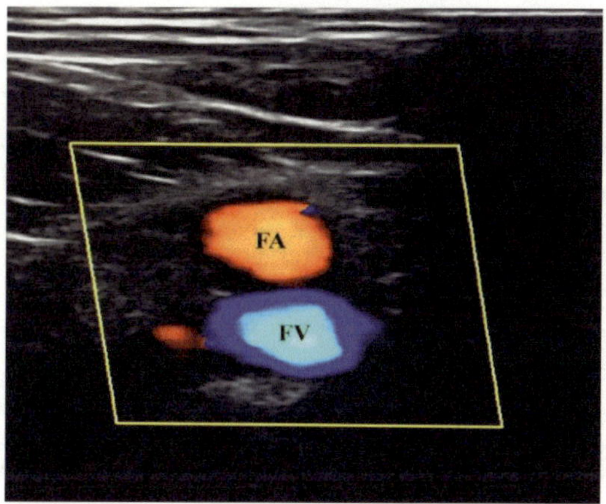

Figure 14. Ultrasound color Doppler imaging of the right femoral artery (FA) and femoral vein (FV). The US probe is installed at a level of 1 cm below the inguinal ligament.

area of the common femoral vein by more than 50% by using head-elevation tilt positions [26]. However, no data on the safety of this maneuver in patients with cardiac arrest and CPR are currently available. First, the femoral vessels in the transverse plane are visualized using a real-time 2D ultrasound, placing an ultrasonic probe under the inguinal ligament. The differentiation between the vein and artery during CPR is performed with a Doppler. The short axis out-of-plane technique is often used for the catheterization of the FV and FA. The long axis in-plane technique is preferable when longitudinal scanning of the femoral vessels is possible. The real-time ultrasound-guided lateral oblique short axis in-plane technique can also be applied. At the same time, no evidence of its preference is available.

Nowadays, femoral vessels are chosen for inserting venoarterial extracorporeal membrane oxygenator devices for extracorporeal CPR and extracorporeal life support [27]. The research results reveal promising outlook of this area of research aimed at saving human life.

6. SV catheterization techniques

The use of a subclavian vein for central venous access during CPR surgery cannot be recommended due to certain limitations. Providing access to the vein may require CPR interruption, and in particular, thorax compression. Besides, a defibrillation electrode may be located in the subclavian area. During CPR, there is a risk of post-puncture pneumo- and hemothorax during SV catheterization. Compared to IJV and FV, the SV anatomical location and its course under the clavicle bone may challenge ultrasound imaging and are accompanied by various artifacts (**Figure 15**).

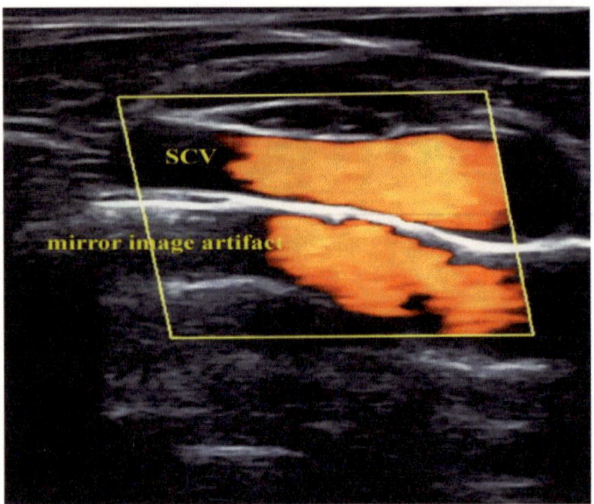

Figure 15. Ultrasound color Doppler imaging of the right subclavian vein (SV) with mirror image artifact.

7. Advantages of ultrasound-guided vascular access during CPR

It can be argued that the use of ultrasound facilitates the identification of the insertion site anatomy, localization of the vessels and their sizes, and differentiating between veins and arteries. Real-time US guidance for puncture allows us to confirm patency of the vessel, as well as needle, wire, and catheter position in the vessel. In addition, ultrasound can be used to determine the change in the filling, and thus, the cross-sectional lumen of the patient, depending on the change in the patient's position (head-down or head-elevation tilt position). In the clinical setting, these advantages allow us to choose the most secure access for puncture and the catheterization of the targeted vessel without interrupting the CPR, reduce the time of intravascular access, minimize the number of unsuccessful catheterization attempts, and reduce the risk of post-puncture complications.

8. Limitations of ultrasound-guided vascular access during CPR

The operator performing ultrasound-guided vascular access is certainly required to have special knowledge and practical skills in visualization of anatomical structures, in particular, blood vessels, during CPR. We assume that anesthesiologists, intensivists, and emergency physicians must be educated about it. To ensure this, special training of operators involved in CVC insertion should be organized. In addition, an intensive care unit must be equipped with US machines to exclude procedural delays. Ultrasound-guided vascular cannulation proved to be effective for cardiopulmonary resuscitation during in-hospital cardiac arrest. This method, however, is not to be recommended during out-of-hospital cardiac arrest, since nowadays there are no data proving its safety and efficiency.

9. Conclusions

Providing satisfactory intravascular access remains an important component of the CPR. Taking into account the advantages of ultrasound-guided central vascular access, it should be considered along with other types of access (peripheral and intraosseous) in patients with in-hospital cardiac arrest.

Conflict of interest

None declared.

Author details

Anton Kasatkin*, Aleksandr Urakov and Anna Nigmatullina

*Address all correspondence to: ant-kasatkin@yandex.ru

Izhevsk State Medical Academy, Izhevsk, Russia

References

[1] Kudenchuk PJ, Cobb LA, Copass MK, Cummins RO, Doherty AM, Fahrenbruch CE, Hallstrom AP, Murray WA, Olsufka M, Walsh T. Amiodarone for resuscitation after out-of-hospital cardiac arrest due to ventricular fibrillation. The New England Journal of Medicine. 1999;**341**:871-878

[2] Rittenberger JC, Menegazzi JJ, Callaway CW. Association of delay to first intervention with return of spontaneous circulation in a swine model of cardiac arrest. Resuscitation. 2007;**73**:154-160

[3] Urakov AL, Kasatkin AA, Urakova NA. Change in local temperature of venous blood and venous vessel walls as a basis for imaging superficial veins during infrared phlebography using temperature-induced tissue contrasting. In: Ng EYK, Etehadtavakol M, editors. Application of Infrared to Biomedical Sciences, Series in BioEngineering. Singapore: Springer Nature Singapore Pte Ltd; 2017. pp. 429-436. DOI: 10.1007/978-981-10-3147-2_24

[4] Ficke BW, Ransom EF, Oakes JE. Near-infrared vein visualization in index finger pollicization. The Journal of Hand Surgery. 2017;**42**(6):481.e1-481.e2. DOI: 10.1016/j.jhsa.2017.03.039

[5] Santos D, Carron PN, Yersin B, Pasquier M. EZ-IO((R)) intraosseous device implementation in a pre-hospital emergency service: A prospective study and review of the literature. Resuscitation. 2013;**84**:440-445

[6] Anson J. A review of intraosseous access in resuscitation. Anesthesiology. 2014;**120**:1015-1031

[7] Brass P, Hellmich M, Kolodziej L, Schick G, Smith AF. Ultrasound guidance versus anatomical landmarks for internal jugular vein catheterization. Cochrane Database of Systematic Reviews. 2015;**9**(1):CD006962. DOI: 10.1002/14651858.CD006962.pub2

[8] Brass P, Hellmich M, Kolodziej L, Schick G, Smith AF. Ultrasound guidance versus anatomical landmarks for subclavian or femoral vein catheterization. Cochrane Database of Systematic Reviews. 2015;**9**(1):CD011447. DOI: 10.1002/14651858.CD011447

[9] Ullman JI, Stoelting RK. Internal jugular vein location with the US Doppler blood flow detector. Anesthesia and Analgesia. 1978;**57**:118. DOI: 10.1213/00000539-197801000-00024

[10] Legler D, Nugent M. Doppler localization of the internal jugular vein facilitates central venous cannulation. Anesthesiology. 1984;**60**(5):481-482

[11] Kawamura R, Okabe M, Namikawa K. Subclavian vein puncture under ultrasonic guidance. Journal of Parenteral and Enteral Nutrition. 1987;**11**(5):505-506

[12] Hilty WM, Hudson PA, Levitt MA, Hall JB. Real-time ultrasound-guided femoral vein catheterization during cardiopulmonary resuscitation. Annals of Emergency Medicine. 1997;**29**(3):331-336

[13] Benassi F, Vezzani A, Vignali L, Gherli T. Ultrasound guided femoral cannulation and percutaneous perfusion of the distal limb for VA ECMO. Journal of Cardiac Surgery. 2014;**29**(3):427-429. DOI: 10.1111/jocs.12319

[14] Troianos CA, Hartman GS, Glas KE, Skubas NJ, Eberhardt RT, Walker JD, Reeves ST. Special articles: Guidelines for performing ultrasound guided vascular cannulation: Recommendations of the American Society of Echocardiography and the Society of Cardiovascular Anesthesiologists. Anesthesia and Analgesia. 2012;**114**:46-72. DOI: 10.1213/ANE.0b013e3182407cd8

[15] Kasatkin AA, Urakov AL, Nigmatullina AR. Using ultrasonography to determine optimal head-down tilt position angle in patients before catheterization of the internal jugular vein. Indian Journal of Critical Care Medicine. 2017;**21**:160-162

[16] Kent A, Patil P, Davila V, Bailey J, Jones C, Evans D, Boulger C, Adkins E, Balakrishnan J, Valiyaveedan S, Galwankar S, Bahner D, Stawicki S. Sonographic evaluation of intravascular volume status: Can internal jugular or femoral vein collapsibility be used in the absence of IVC visualization? Annals of Thoracic Medicine. 2015;**10**(1):44-49. DOI: 10.4103/1817-1737.146872

[17] Dietrich CF, Horn R, Morf S, Chiorean L, Dong Y, Cui XW, Atkinson NS, Jenssen C. Ultrasound-guided central vascular interventions, comments on the European Federation of Societies for Ultrasound in Medicine and Biology guidelines on interventional ultrasound. Journal of Thoracic Disease. 2016;**8**:E851-E868. DOI: 10.21037/jtd.2016.08.49

[18] Denys BG, Uretsky BF. Anatomical variations of internal jugular vein location: Impact on central venous access. Critical Care Medicine. 1991;**19**:1516-1519

[19] Denys BG, Uretsky BF, Reddy PS. Ultrasound-assisted cannulation of the internal jugular vein. A prospective comparison to the external landmark-guided technique. Circulation. 1993;**87**:1557-1562

[20] Gallieni M, Martina V, Rizzo MA. Central venous catheters: Legal issues. The Journal of Vascular Access. 2011;**12**:273-279

[21] Rossi UG, Dahmane M, Petrocelli F, Patrone L, Gola G, Ferro C. Comparison between vertical and lateral ultrasound-guided technique for percutaneous internal jugular venous cannulation in permanent central venous access. Cardiovascular and Interventional Radiology. 2012;**35**:S211

[22] Rossi U, Rigamonti P, Tichà V, Zoffoli E, Giordano A, Gallieni M, Cariati M. Percutaneous ultrasound-guided central venous catheters: The lateral in-plane technique for internal jugular vein access. The Journal of Vascular Access. 2014;**15**(1):56-60. DOI: 10.5301/jva.5000177

[23] Mey U, Glasmacher A, Hahn C, et al. Evaluation of an ultrasound-guided technique for central venous access via the internal jugular vein in 493 patients. Support Care Cancer. 2003;**11**(3):148-155

[24] Kasatkin A, Nigmatullina A, Urakov A, Shchegolev A. Method for internal jugular catheterisation by lateral access. RU Patent 2,655,449. 2018

[25] Werner SL, Jones RA, Emerman CL. Effect of hip abduction and external rotation on femoral vein exposure for possible cannulation. The Journal of Emergency Medicine. 2008;**35**:73-75

[26] Hopkins JW, Warkentine F, Gracely E, Kim IK. The anatomic relationship between the femoral artery and common femoral vein in frog leg position versus straight leg position in pediatric patients. Academic Emergency Medicine. 2009;**16**:579-584

[27] Mosier J, Kelsey M, Raz Y, Gunnerson K, Meyer R, Hypes C, Malo J, Whitmore S, Spaite D. Extracorporeal membrane oxygenation (ECMO) for critically ill adults in the emergency department: History, current applications, and future directions. Critical Care. 2015;**19**:431. DOI: 10.1186/s13054-015-1155-7

Chapter 5

Applications of the Transthoracic Impedance Signal during Resuscitation

Digna M. González-Otero, Sofía Ruiz de Gauna, José Julio Gutiérrez, Purificación Saiz and Jesus M. Ruiz

Additional information is available at the end of the chapter

http://dx.doi.org/10.5772/intechopen.79382

Abstract

Defibrillators acquire both the ECG and the transthoracic impedance (TI) signal through defibrillation pads. TI represents the resistance of the thorax to current flow, and is measured by defibrillators to check that defibrillation pads are correctly attached to the chest of the patient. Additionally, some defibrillators use the TI measurement to adjust the energy of the defibrillation pulse. Changes in tissue composition due to redistribution and movement of fluids induce fluctuations in the TI. Blood flow during the cardiac cycle generates small fluctuations synchronized to each heartbeat. Respiration (or assisted ventilation) also causes changes in the TI. Additionally, during cardiopulmonary resuscitation (CPR), chest compressions cause a disturbance in the electrode-skin interface, inducing artifacts in the TI signal. These fluctuations may provide useful information regarding CPR quality, length of pauses in chest compressions (no flow time), presence of circulation, etc. This chapter explores the new applications of the transthoracic impedance signal acquired through defibrillation pads during resuscitative attempts.

Keywords: transthoracic impedance, defibrillator, cardiac arrest, ventilation rate, chest compression rate, circulation detection

1. Introduction

Biological tissues strongly differ in terms of their electrical impedance. For instance, the resistivities of blood, cardiac muscle, and lungs are 150, 750, and 1275 Ω/cm, respectively [1]. This variability makes the measurement of electric impedance useful in understanding the functioning and viability of internal organs. In fact, impedance plethysmography, a

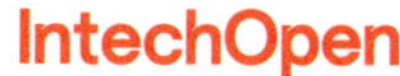

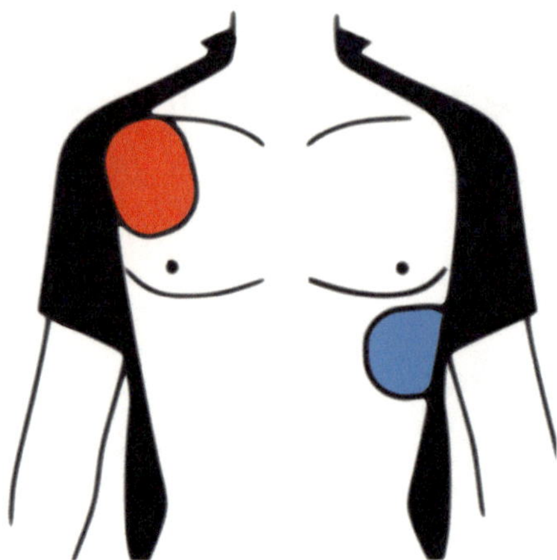

Figure 1. Anterolateral position for self-adhesive defibrillation pads. Source: Bexen Cardio.

well-established technique to determine changing tissue volumes based on the measurement of electric impedance at the body surface, is widely used for multiple applications, including the measurement of lung water content, the diagnosis of deep venous thrombosis, and the determination of cardiac stroke volume.

In the field of resuscitation, transthoracic impedance (TI) is measured by defibrillators through defibrillation pads, together with the ECG signal. **Figure 1** shows the recommended anterolateral position for the defibrillation pads, with one pad placed below the right clavicle and the other one below the left axilla. TI represents the resistance of the thorax to current flow, and can be measured by passing an alternate current through the tissue and measuring the induced voltage drop.

Defibrillators, particularly automated external defibrillators (AEDs), measure the TI to check that the defibrillation pads are correctly attached to the chest of the patient. TI is approximately 70–80Ω in adults, but it varies considerably between subjects, with a range of 15–150Ω [2, 3]. Baseline TI is affected by several factors including chest size, distance between the electrodes, electrode size, and the interface between the electrodes and the chest wall [4]. Too high impedance values indicate that the contact between the pads and the skin is inadequate. A good skin-electrode contact is critical for a safe delivery of the electrical shock and for a correct ECG acquisition, essential for a reliable rhythm analysis. AEDs monitor the TI signal and guide the rescuer through the resuscitation process. Typical AED messages prompt rescuers to attach the electrodes to the chest of the patient, to check the contact between the electrodes and the skin if the measured impedance is inadequate, or to avoid touching the patient during AED rhythm assessment.

Additionally, some defibrillators use the TI measurement to adjust the energy of the defibrillation pulse (impedance compensation technique) [5, 6]. Successful defibrillation requires that sufficient current flows through the heart muscle, but excessive current during electrical shock may cause myocardial damage. Thus, shocks should be provided with the lowest amount of energy that will achieve defibrillation. However, the actual current flow is determined not only by the selected energy but also by the TI of the patient. An energy level that is adequate

http://dx.doi.org/10.5772/intechopen.79382

for a low-impedance patient may not achieve defibrillation in a patient with higher impedance. Modern biphasic defibrillators measure TI and adjust the energy delivery accordingly.

These two applications of the TI signal in defibrillators rely on its baseline value. However, as in the impedance plethysmography, changes in tissue composition due to redistribution and movement of fluids induce fluctuations in the TI acquired through defibrillation pads. During the cardiac cycle, the distribution and amount of blood in the thorax varies, causing small changes in the conductivity of the tissue that are reflected in the TI waveform [7]. Respiration (or ventilation of the patient) also affects TI; impedance increases during inspiration and decreases again during expiration [8]. Additionally, during cardiopulmonary resuscitation (CPR), chest compressions cause a disturbance in the electrode-skin interface, inducing artifacts in the ECG and in the TI signal [9].

This chapter explores the new applications of the TI signal acquired through defibrillation pads derived from the analysis of these variations.

2. Transthoracic impedance for circulation detection

Previous releases of basic life support (BLS) resuscitation guidelines recommended assessing if the patient presented signs of circulation by checking the carotid pulse before starting chest compressions. However, several studies have shown that pulse palpation is time-consuming and inaccurate not only for lay rescuers with basic CPR training [10], but also for healthcare professionals [11]. Based on the existing evidence, resuscitation guidelines removed the pulse check recommendation for laypeople in their 2000 release. However, reliable identification of pulse-generating rhythms would be useful to distinguish cardiac arrest from other collapse states, and to detect the return of spontaneous circulation during a resuscitative attempt.

Circulation induces low-amplitude fluctuations in the TI. **Figure 2** shows an example of the fluctuations induced with each heartbeat for a patient presenting a pulse-generating rhythm. Top panels show the ECG of the patient in mV, and the bottom panel the corresponding TI signal in Ohms (Ω). Several authors have studied the potential of the TI signal to reliably detect the presence of circulation.

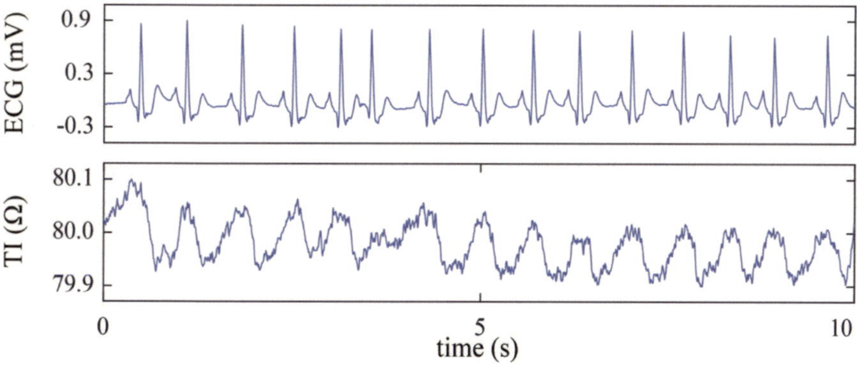

Figure 2. Fluctuations induced by circulation in the TI.

2.1. State of the art

Back in 1998, Johnston et al. showed that the TI acquired through defibrillation pads could be potentially used to discriminate between pulse-generating rhythms and those associated with hemodynamic collapse [7]. Using recordings acquired during cardiac arrest episodes, they extracted four features from the TI signal and evaluated their ability to identify pulse-generating rhythms. Their results were promising, and they suggested using this method to increase the sensitivity of shock advice algorithms in AEDs.

Four years later, Pellis et al. [12] showed in a laboratory study with anesthetized swine that the TI signal measured through defibrillation pads presented fluctuations coincident with cardiac contraction, and larger and slower fluctuations coincident with ventilations. After inducing VF to the animals, all the fluctuations ceased. The authors proposed equipping AEDs with cardiac and respiratory arrest detectors based on the analysis of the TI.

Later, in 2007, Losert et al. proposed a classifier based on neural networks to detect the return of spontaneous circulation during the resuscitative attempt [8]. They extracted several features derived from the circulatory-related waveform of the TI, and evaluated the performance of the classifier using recordings collected from hemodynamically stable and cardiac arrest patients. With their dataset, they could identify patients presenting an arterial blood pressure above 80 mmHg with a sensitivity of 90% and a specificity of 82%.

The following year, Risdal et al. introduced a new classifier based on pattern recognition to discriminate between pulseless electrical activity and pulsatile rhythms [13]. The method used clinical data, and presented a sensitivity and specificity for the detection of pulse-generating rhythms of 91 and 90%, respectively. That same year, Cromie et al. showed in an animal model that the Fast Fourier Transform (FFT) of the impedance cardiogram recorded through defibrillation pads was a potential clinical marker of cardiac arrest [14]. In a subsequent clinical study, they refined the method and evaluated its performance with in-hospital cardiac arrest and nonarrest patients [15]. They concluded that selective filtering of the impedance cardiogram was a powerful hemodynamic sensor of cardiac arrest, with a sensitivity (specificity) of 81% (97%) in the validation set. In 2012, Krasteva et al. showed that the TI recorded through defibrillation pads during cardioversion provides information about the quality of myocardial contraction associated to sinus rhythm, asystole, and different arrhythmias [16, 17].

More recently, in 2013, Ruiz and coauthors postulated that the circulation component of the TI signal acquired through defibrillation pads could be reliably isolated [18]. They proposed an adaptive system based on a least mean square algorithm that used detected QRS complexes as a reference to extract the circulation component of the TI, and obtained several features from the circulation component and its first derivative. When trying to discriminate between pulseless electrical activity and pulsatile rhythms in cardiac arrest victims, all features showed an area under the curve (AUC) higher than 0.96. Later, Alonso et al. proposed another adaptive method, also using the QRS instants as a reference to extract the TI circulation component [19]. They designed a classifier between pulsatile rhythm and pulseless electrical activity based on a multivariate logistic regression model than included six features extracted from the ECG and from the TI signals. When evaluated with recordings acquired by monitor-defibrillators during advanced life support, they reported a sensitivity (specificity) in the detection of pulsatile rhythms of 92% (92%).

Although several authors have proved that the TI signal recorded by AEDs contains information regarding blood circulation, isolating its circulation component may be challenging. Chest compressions and ventilations induce fluctuations in the TI signal, with amplitudes higher than those attributable to cardiac contraction. In addition, because of the noise caused by patient movement or inadequate electrode-skin contact, the TI signal may become unreliable. To address these challenges, in a later study, Ruiz et al. proposed launching an automated assessment of blood circulation during AED rhythm analysis intervals [20]. Their hypothesis was that, as during those segments nobody should be touching the patient, the ECG and TI signals would not be affected by chest compressions, ventilations, or patient movement, and thus, the algorithm would be more reliable. Additionally, they proposed a very simple method that could be implemented in current AEDs. When evaluated with AED recordings obtained from out-of-hospital cardiac arrest interventions, their method reported a sensitivity (specificity) for detecting pulsatile rhythms of 98% (98%). The authors suggested how the circulation detection algorithm could be included in the AED sequence. After rhythm analysis, in case a nonshockable nonasystole rhythm is detected, the circulation detection algorithm should be launched to assess if the underlying rhythm corresponds to a pulsatile rhythm or to pulseless electrical activity. If circulation is detected, the responder should check if the patient is responsive and breathing normally to confirm the return of spontaneous circulation. If after 10 s the rescuer cannot confirm the presence of circulation, CPR should be resumed.

2.2. Discussion

AEDs are very reliable in detecting malignant arrhythmias, but they cannot distinguish between pulsatile rhythms and pulseless electrical activity. When a nonshockable rhythm is identified, rescuers are prompted to resume CPR, even if the patient has recovered spontaneous circulation.

Since the removal of the pulse check recommendation for laypeople in resuscitation guidelines, several studies have explored the possibility of expanding the functionality of conventional AEDs to reliably detect the presence of circulation. It is widely accepted that the TI signal contains useful information for the identification of pulse-generating rhythms. Some of the published studies suggest launching the circulation detector while the AED is performing a rhythm analysis. This would maximize signal quality, as artifact induced by chest compressions, ventilations, or by patient movement would be avoided. Although some of the proposed methods are complex and computationally expensive, others are much simpler, which lowers the barrier to implementation.

The use of enhanced AEDs able to detect circulation could help BLS providers to confirm cardiac arrest and to identify the return of spontaneous circulation, which would avoid unnecessarily prolonging CPR. However, further validation is still required for the clinical implementation of these methods.

3. Transthoracic impedance for ventilation detection

Medical treatment of cardiac arrest involves early CPR and early defibrillation. Resuscitation guidelines [21] recommend providing chest compressions and ventilations with a 30:2 ratio before intubation and continuous chest compressions with a ventilation rate of 8–12 per minute afterward. Unfortunately, hyperventilation is common both in hospital and out of hospital [22, 23]. In animal studies, these excessive ventilation rates resulted in decreased coronary perfusion pressures and poor outcomes [24, 25], although some conflicting results have been presented [26].

Respiration and ventilation of the patient induce fluctuations in the TI signal acquired by defibrillators; impedance increases about 0.2–3Ω during inspiration and decreases again during expiration. Mainly, two effects cause these changes: first, during inspiration, there is an increase in the gas volume of the chest in relation to the fluid volume, which causes conductivity to decrease; additionally, during inspiration, the distance between the electrode pads increases because of chest expansion, which also increases resistance.

Figures 3 and **4** illustrate this effect for a patient presenting return of spontaneous circulation and for a cardiac arrest patient who is receiving CPR, respectively. In **Figure 3**, fluctuations induced by circulation and by respiration are observed in the second panel. The baseline impedance of the patient is about 103Ω, but, during inspiration, the impedance value increases between 1 and 2Ω. In this segment, eight breaths are distinguished. The patient presented a pulse-generating rhythm, confirmed by fast and low-amplitude fluctuations in the TI of approximately 0.2Ω, synchronized with every QRS complex; this is the circulatory component of the TI.

Figure 4 shows a segment of the compression depth and TI signals recorded during a resuscitation episode while the patient was receiving 30:2 CPR. In this segment, 4 series of 15 compressions can be observed, with pauses in between for ventilation. Each compression induced a fluctuation in the TI, with a peak-to-peak amplitude of almost 4Ω in this case. During each pause, the patient was ventilated twice, and slower fluctuations were induced in the TI.

The analysis of the TI acquired through defibrillation pads could be useful for ventilation monitoring, either in real time, to guide rescuers during the resuscitation event, or for episode

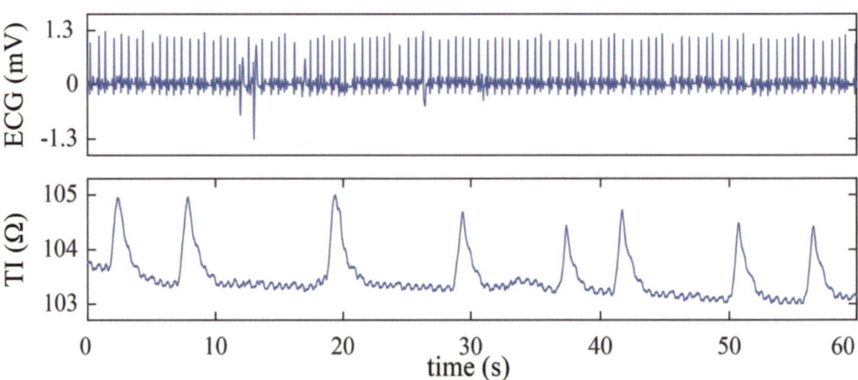

Figure 3. Segment of TI signal with circulatory and respiration-related components.

http://dx.doi.org/10.5772/intechopen.79382

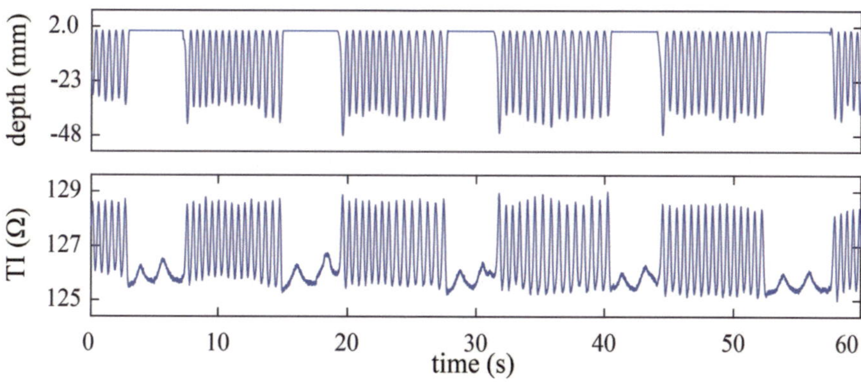

Figure 4. Segment of TI signal with artifact induced by chest compressions and fluctuations induced by ventilations.

debriefing afterward. However, the amplitude and duration of the TI fluctuations vary widely along the resuscitation episode and among different patients. Moreover, patient movement and chest compressions induce artifacts in the TI, which complicate the identification of the fluctuations induced by ventilations, especially when compressions and ventilations are applied simultaneously, as in the case of intubated patients.

3.1. State of the art

Pellis et al. were the first to suggest the ability of the TI signal acquired by defibrillators to determine the presence or absence of breathing, back in 2002 [12]. In an experiment with anesthetized swine, they found that the TI signal acquired through conventional defibrillation electrodes showed large fluctuations time coincident with the ventilations identified in the capnogram.

In 2006, Losert et al. performed a clinical study to investigate the potential of the TI measured via defibrillator pads for measuring ventilation rate and inspiration time [8]. They selected a convenience sample of mechanical ventilated patients, cardiac arrest patients and patients after restoration of spontaneous circulation, and calculated the correlation in waveform between TI and tidal volume given by a ventilator. The median correlation between the impedance waveform and the tidal volume waveform was 0.97 for all patient groups. They concluded that the TI provides information regarding tidal volumes when chest compressions are interrupted, and that it can be useful to quantify ventilation rates and inspiration times.

The following year, Risdal et al. proposed the first automated system to detect ventilation during ongoing CPR by analyzing the TI signal [27]. They developed a pattern-recognition-based detector and used recordings of resuscitation efforts to train it and to evaluate its performance. The annotated ventilations were detected with a sensitivity of 90% and a positive predictive value of 96%. Although the results were good, the method demanded high computational resources, which could limit its practical implementation.

Kramer-Johansen et al. used the TI signal to annotate ventilations in a clinical study about CPR quality before and after endotracheal intubation [28]. In 3% of the episodes, the fluctuations induced by ventilations in the TI signal disappeared after placing the endotracheal tube.

The authors suspected that this was due to accidental esophageal intubation and hypothesized that analysis of the TI could be used to identify incorrect tube placement. Two years later, in a prospective clinical study [29], they confirmed that the TI was useful to detect misplaced endotracheal tubes. With a dataset of 123 esophageal and 178 tracheal ventilations, tube position was predicted with a sensitivity of 99% and a specificity of 97%.

More recently, in 2010, Edelson et al. developed and compared the performance of two methods to detect ventilations during CPR, one of them based on the TI signal and the other one based on the capnogram [30]. They concluded that both methods underestimated ventilation rate, and suggested that the optimal strategy could be combining them. The TI-based detector underestimated ventilation rate because of artifacts induced in the TI signal during chest compressions and patient movement and because low-amplitude ventilations generated too small fluctuations.

González-Otero et al. presented in a conference paper in 2013 a simple impedance-based method for ventilation detection during CPR [31]. Their aim was to develop a method to be implemented in AEDs for ventilation rate monitoring. The detection algorithm first identified fluctuations in the preprocessed TI signal. Then, it characterized the fluctuations by features of amplitude, duration, and slope. Finally, a decision system based on thresholds was applied to decide whether each fluctuation corresponded to a ventilation. When evaluated with out-of-hospital cardiac arrest records, the algorithm presented a sensitivity and positive predictive value of 97 and 95%, respectively.

In 2015, Alonso et al. combined a simple impedance-based method to identify ventilations in the TI with a method to identify chest compressions [32]. Their aim was to evaluate the accuracy and reliability of the TI signal to assess CPR quality metrics. Their combined detector provided good results with out-of-hospital cardiac arrest records, with a sensitivity and positive predictive value of 98 and 81% for ventilation detection.

3.2. Discussion

Respiration and assisted ventilation induce fluctuations in the TI signal acquired through defibrillation pads. Several authors have analyzed the ability of this signal to identify ventilations, and concluded that the TI is an indicator of ventilation rate. However, the technology is not perfect. The main challenges to be addressed are that low-volume ventilations usually generate low-amplitude fluctuations difficult to detect, and that patient movement and chest compressions induce artifact in the TI signal that complicate ventilation detection. Although artifact induced by chest compressions can be suppressed using filtering techniques, residuals in the filtered TI signal may induce errors in the ventilation detection process.

Figure 5 shows two examples of the TI signal before and after being filtered for ventilation detection using the technique described in [31]. In example (a), the patient received six ventilations (depicted with vertical red lines), the first two overlapped with chest compressions. After the filtering process, the artifact induced by chest compressions was suppressed, and the ventilations could be correctly identified. In example (b), the onset and the offset of the chest compression interval altered the filtered TI and induced fluctuations that were incorrectly identified as ventilations (false positives).

http://dx.doi.org/10.5772/intechopen.79382

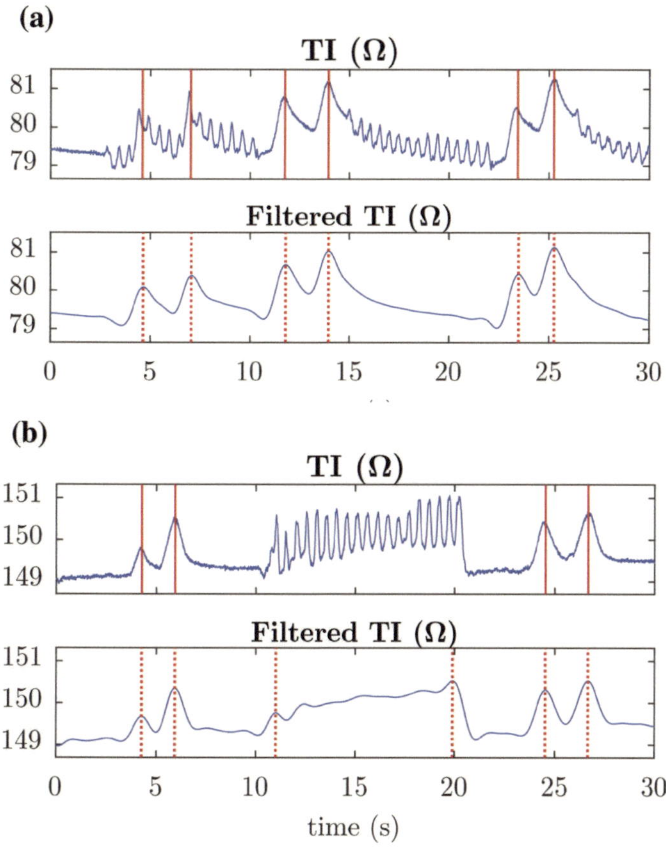

Figure 5. Examples of TI signal before and after being filtered for ventilation detection. Example (a) illustrates correct ventilation identifications, while example (b) illustrates false-positive detections.

Although there is still room for improvement, it is widely accepted that the TI signal is a reliable indicator of ventilation rate, and a good option when no other signal such as capnography is available for ventilation monitoring. In fact, various commercial AEDs analyze the TI in real time to provide feedback to the rescuer regarding ventilation rate during the resuscitative attempt. Additionally, some manufacturers use the TI signal to compute ventilation rate in offline applications for episode debriefing.

4. Transthoracic impedance for chest compression characterization

Resuscitation guidelines emphasize the importance of providing high-quality chest compressions during CPR, that is, compressions with an adequate rate and depth, completely releasing the chest after each compression, and minimizing interruptions [21]. During CPR, chest compressions induce fluctuations in the TI. These fluctuations are caused both by true variations in the impedance value associated to the thoracic volume change and by motion artifact induced by the disruption of the electrode-skin interface. Several researchers have investigated the feasibility of using the TI signal to extract information about chest compressions during CPR. Some of the proposed applications include identification of chest compression pauses, calculation of chest compression rate, and estimation of chest compression depth. The following sections present an overview of the state of the art in those three topics.

4.1. Automated detection of pauses in chest compressions

Interruptions in chest compressions are frequent during out-of-hospital cardiac arrest. Following current resuscitation guidelines, chest compressions are interrupted for assisted ventilation (BLS sequence), to assess the rhythm, to defibrillate, and to change rescuers. These interruptions compromise the blood flow to the heart and brain and have an adverse effect on defibrillation success, and, consequently, on survival [33, 34].

The automated detection of pauses in chest compressions would be relevant for two main reasons. First, in the field of CPR quality, it would enable AEDs to provide feedback to the rescuer when too long interruptions in chest compressions are detected. Second, it would allow detecting CPR artifact-free ECG intervals (for example, pauses for ventilation of the patient or rescuer switch) in which the AEDs could reliably assess the ECG rhythm, without requiring an additional interruption of chest compressions for rhythm assessment.

Chest compressions and ventilations induce fast and slow fluctuations in the TI signal, respectively. In 2012, González-Otero et al. published in a conference proceedings a simple method for the automated detection of pauses in chest compressions using the TI acquired by defibrillators [35]. **Figure 6** illustrates the application of the method. The fluctuations induced by chest compressions (first panel) are first isolated by applying a filter that suppresses the fluctuations induced by ventilations. The result of this filtering process is shown in the second panel. Then, chest compressions are emphasized by computing the slope of the signal as the first difference, scaled and squared (third panel). Finally, the fluctuations are smoothed by applying a first-order low-pass filter of a cutoff frequency of 0.6 Hz, and using an adaptive threshold, the intervals without chest compressions are identified (fourth panel). A small delay correction is applied to the detected onset and offset of the chest compression pauses to compensate the delay introduced by the process.

The performance of this method was evaluated using 600 out-of-hospital cardiac arrest records. In the test database, sensitivity and positive predictive value for the detection of pauses in chest compressions were 93.9 and 96.2%, respectively. The difference between the durations of the detected and of the annotated pauses was 0.24 ± 0.73 s.

Some AEDs implement similar algorithms to identify too long pauses in chest compressions, and to prompt the rescuer to resume CPR. Additionally, the detected pauses, which are free of motion artifact induced by chest compressions, could be used by AEDs to launch a rhythm analysis, avoiding additional interruptions in chest compressions, as proposed by Ruiz de Gauna et al. in 2012 [36]. In 2013, Ruiz et al. analyzed the accuracy of a fast shock advice algorithm able to provide a shock/no shock decision in 3 s when it was launched during chest compression pauses [37]. Their algorithm was evaluated with 110 shockable and 466 non-shockable segments extracted from 235 out-of-hospital cardiac arrest episodes. This dataset

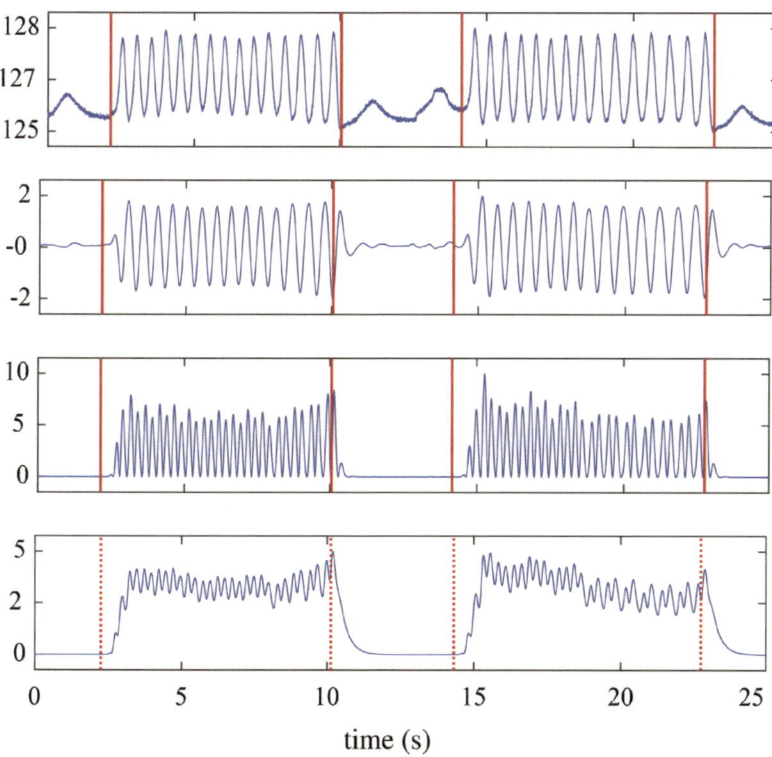

Figure 6. Signals involved in the chest compression pauses detection method described by González-Otero et al. [34].

comprised 4476 pauses, 2183 of them containing two ventilations. A total of 92% of the pauses and 95% of the pauses with two ventilations were long enough to launch the shock advice algorithm. The overall sensitivity and specificity of the shock advice algorithm for the detection of shockable rhythms were 96 and 97%, respectively.

When CPR is provided at the standard 30:2 compression-ventilation ratio, this method would allow the AED to diagnose the rhythm after each series of 30 chest compressions, that is, approximately every 20 s. Current resuscitation guidelines recommend interrupting CPR every 2 min for rhythm assessment. These preshock pauses would be eliminated by analyzing the rhythm during ventilation pauses. Additionally, a rhythm assessment would be performed every 20 s instead of every 2 min, so more information regarding rhythm evolution would be available. This could potentially be useful to guide the therapy, for example, by early recognition of recurrent ventricular fibrillation.

4.2. Chest compression rate estimation

Resuscitation guidelines recommend providing chest compressions at a rate between 100 and 120 compressions per minute (cpm) during CPR. Two studies found higher survival among patients that received compressions at those rates compared to those who received slower or faster compressions [38, 39]. Additionally, very high chest compression rates were associated with reduced compression depths, which are detrimental to survival. However, studies on CPR quality have shown that providing high-quality chest compressions is challenging both for laypeople and for well-trained rescuers [40].

The use of metronomes and real-time CPR feedback devices can improve adherence to CPR quality guidelines [41]. Metronomes generate regular audible beats that help rescuers to follow a rhythm, for example, recommended compression rate. Feedback systems are more sophisticated, and measure CPR performance in real time [42, 43]. Most of them are accessory devices that are placed between the hands of the rescuer and the chest of the patient during CPR. This adds complexity to the equipment and limits the widespread of feedback systems, particularly in BLS settings.

Chest compressions induce fluctuations in the TI signal. Analyzing these fluctuations could be a simple way to monitor chest compression rate without requiring additional devices. Several authors [32, 44–47] have suggested using the TI signal to compute chest compression rate either online, to provide feedback to the rescuer during a resuscitation attempt, or offline, for episode debriefing.

The main challenge in computing compression rate from the TI signal derives from the fact that an important component of the fluctuations induced in the TI is an artifact generated in the electrode-skin interface. As an artifact, its characteristics are influenced by many factors including the TI acquisition front-end, the electrode type, the stiffness of the patient's chest and CPR performance (rate, depth, applied force and acceleration). **Figure 7** shows two segments of TI signals acquired by different defibrillators with different TI acquisition front-ends. In both segments, the chest compressions were provided at a similar rate (about 100 cpm). However, in example (a), the fluctuations induced in the TI signal were quite sinusoidal, while in example (b), they had a very strong second harmonic component, causing a distinct waveform.

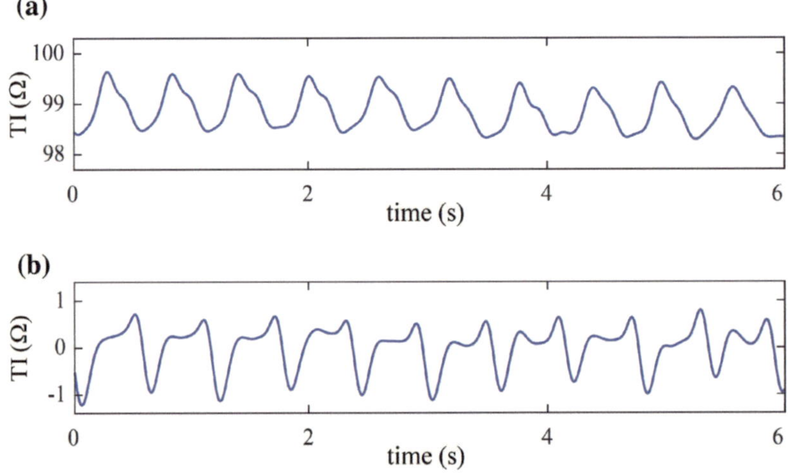

Figure 7. TI signals obtained from two different defibrillators during chest compressions.

Most of the methods to compute compression rate from the TI signal that have been published in the literature were optimized and tested with subsets obtained from a single monitor-defibrillator, and thus the variability introduced by the signal acquisition front-end was not taken into account. A later study [47] presented a general method to calculate chest compression rate, and evaluated its accuracy with three different databases of out-of-hospital cardiac arrest records. The authors concluded that it is possible to reliably estimate compression rate by processing the TI, although the performance of the method will vary with the characteristics of the TI fluctuations.

Methods to measure compression rate based on the TI signal are being commercially used both in applications for episode debriefing and in defibrillators to provide feedback to the rescuers in real time.

4.3. Chest compression depth estimation

Feedback devices can be used during CPR to guide chest compression depth and improve CPR quality, but this implies using an additional device [42]. Some authors suggested that fluctuations induced in the TI could be a potential indicator of compression depth [48, 49]. Unfortunately, those studies were published in short communications, and details on the analytical methods and the datasets used were not provided. In 2012, Zhang et al. investigated the relationship between TI fluctuations and compression depth in an animal study [50]. Two experts provided chest compressions with different depths, suboptimal (35 mm) and optimal (50 mm), to 14 anesthetized swine. They evaluated the correlation between the peak-through amplitude of the fluctuations induced in the TI during chest compressions and the compression depth, and found a high correlation (Pearson correlation coefficient $r = 0.89$). Additionally, they found great differences in TI amplitude between optimal and suboptimal depth groups. These results were promising, and suggested that TI could be useful for monitoring compression depth.

Two years later, Alonso et al. [51] studied the correlation of TI with compression depth using a large database of out-of-hospital cardiac arrest recordings. They extracted three morphologic features of the TI signal and analyzed their correlation with compression depth. This correlation was evaluated for the whole population, for each patient individually, and for segments corresponding to a single patient and a single rescuer. Additionally, trying to replicate the experiments of Zhang et al., they included the correlation when only series of optimal or suboptimal chest compressions (no intermediate values) were included. In their study, the prediction of compression depth based on any of the morphologic features of the TI was highly unreliable. When only optimal and suboptimal chest compressions were included, the correlation coefficient increased, but there was still a high variability. The authors concluded that when a wide variety of patients and rescuers are included, chest compression depth could not be reliably estimated from features extracted from the TI signal.

5. Conclusions

The TI signal is potentially available in any resuscitation attempt in which adhesive defibrillation pads are used. This signal was customarily acquired to check if the defibrillation pads were correctly attached to the chest of the patient and to adjust the energy of the defibrillating shock. In the last years, new applications have been suggested. Respiration (or assisted ventilation), changes in blood flow during the cardiac cycle, and chest compressions induce fluctuations in the TI. By analyzing these fluctuations, useful information can be extracted regarding CPR quality and patient status. Some of these new applications, such as TI-based ventilation rate and chest compression rate computation, have been thoroughly validated and are implemented in AEDs or in offline programs for episode debriefing. Other applications, such as circulation detection, require further studies before clinical use. Finally, with the current technology, compression depth cannot be accurately computed from the TI signal. In any case, the TI signal has the potential to serve as a real-time noninvasive indicator of CPR quality and of patient status, and has the advantage of being widely available.

Acknowledgements

This research received financial support from the Spanish Government through the project TEC2012-31144 and from the Basque Government through the grant BFI-2011-166 and through the project IT1087-16.

Some sections of this book chapter are related to the thesis work *Feedback systems for the quality of chest compressions during cardiopulmonary resuscitation* carried out by coauthor Digna M. González-Otero, under the supervision of coauthors Jesus Ruiz and Sofía Ruiz de Gauna [43]. Several parts of this work have been published in indexed journals or presented at international conferences.

Conflict of interest

No potential conflict of interest was reported by the authors.

Author details

Digna M. González-Otero*, Sofía Ruiz de Gauna, José Julio Gutiérrez, Purificación Saiz and Jesus M. Ruiz

*Address all correspondence to: dignamaria.gonzalez@ehu.eus

University of the Basque Country (UPV/EHU), Bilbao, Spain

References

[1] Baker LE. Principles of the impedance technique. IEEE Engineering in Medicine and Biology Magazine. 1989;8(1):11-15

[2] Kerber RE, Grayzel J, Hoyt R, Marcus M, Kennedy J. Transthoracic resistance in human defibrillation. Influence of body weight, chest size, serial shocks, paddle size and paddle contact pressure. Circulation. 1981;**63**(3):676-682

[3] Kerber RE, Kouba C, Martins J, Kelly K, Low R, Hoyt R, et al. Advance prediction of transthoracic impedance in human defibrillation and cardioversion: Importance of impedance in determining the success of low-energy shocks. Circulation. 1984;**70**(2):303-308

[4] Kerber RE, Deakin CD, Tacker WA Jr. Transthoracic defibrillation. In: Paradir NA, Halperin HR, Kern KB, Wenzel V, Chamberlain D, editors. Cardiac Arrest: Science and Practice of Resuscitation Medicine. Cambridge: Cambridge University Press; 2007. pp. 470-481

[5] Kerber RE, Martins J, Kienzle M, Constantin L, Olshansky B, Hopson R, et al. Energy, current, and success in defibrillation and cardioversion: Clinical studies using an automated impedance-based method of energy adjustment. Circulation. 1988;**77**(5):1038-1046

[6] Li Y, Ristagno G, Yu T, Bisera J, Weil MH, Tang W. A comparison of defibrillation efficacy between different impedance compensation techniques in high impedance porcine model. Resuscitation. 2009;**80**(11):1312-1317

[7] Johnston PW, Imam Z, Dempsey G, Anderson J, Adgey AA. The transthoracic impedance cardiogram is a potential haemodynamic sensor for an automated external defibrillator. European Heart Journal. 1998;**19**(12):1879-1888

[8] Losert H, Risdal M, Sterz F, Nysaether J, Köhler K, Eftestøl T, et al. Thoracic impedance changes measured via defibrillator pads can monitor ventilation in critically ill patients and during cardiopulmonary resuscitation. Critical Care Medicine. 2006;**34**(9):2399-2405

[9] Fitzgibbon E, Berger R, Tsitlik J, Halperin HR. Determination of the noise source in the electrocardiogram during cardiopulmonary resuscitation. Critical Care Medicine. 2002;**30**(4):S148-S153

[10] Eberle B, Dick WF, Schneider T, Wisser G, Doetsch S, Tzanova I. Checking the carotid pulse check: Diagnostic accuracy of first responders in patients with and without a pulse. Resuscitation. 1996;**33**(2):107-116

[11] Tibballs J, Weeranatna C. The influence of time on the accuracy of healthcare personnel to diagnose paediatric cardiac arrest by pulse palpation. Resuscitation. 2010;**81**(6):671-675

[12] Pellis T, Bisera J, Tang W, Weil MH. Expanding automatic external defibrillators to include automated detection of cardiac, respiratory, and cardiorespiratory arrest. Critical Care Medicine. 2002;**30**(4):S176-S178

[13] Risdal M, Aase SO, Kramer-Johansen J, Eftestol T. Automatic identification of return of spontaneous circulation during cardiopulmonary resuscitation. IEEE Transactions on Biomedical Engineering. 2008;**55**(1):60-68

[14] Cromie NA, Allen JD, Turner C, Anderson JM, Adgey AAJ. The impedance cardiogram recorded through two electrocardiogram/defibrillator pads as a determinant of cardiac arrest during experimental studies. Critical Care Medicine. 2008;**36**(5):1578-1584

[15] Cromie NA, Allen JD, Navarro C, Turner C, Anderson JM, Adgey AAJ. Assessment of the impedance cardiogram recorded by an automated external defibrillator during clinical cardiac arrest. Critical Care Medicine. 2010;**38**(2):510-517

[16] Krasteva V, Jekova I, Trendafilova E, Ménétré S, Mudrov T, Didon JP. Study of transthoracic impedance cardiogram for assessment of cardiac hemodynamics in atrial fibrillation patents. International Journal Bioautomation. 2012;**16**(3):203-210

[17] Krasteva V, Jekova I, Trendafilova E, Ménétré S, Mudrov TN, Didon JP. Transthoracic impedance cardiogram indicates for compromised cardiac hemodynamics in different supraventricular and ventricular arrhythmias. Annual Journal of Electronics. 2012;**6**(1): 23-26

[18] Ruiz J, Alonso E, Aramendi E, Kramer-Johansen J, Eftestøl T, Ayala U, et al. Reliable extraction of the circulation component in the thoracic impedance measured by defibrillation pads. Resuscitation. 2013;**84**(10):1345-1352

[19] Alonso E, Aramendi E, Daya M, Irusta U, Chicote B, Russell JK, et al. Circulation detection using the electrocardiogram and the thoracic impedance acquired by defibrillation pads. Resuscitation. 2016;**99**:56-62

[20] Ruiz J, Ruiz de Gauna S, González-Otero DM, Saiz P, Gutiérrez JJ, Veintemillas JF, et al. Circulation assessment by automated external defibrillators during cardiopulmonary resuscitation. Resuscitation. 2018;**128**:158-163

[21] Perkins GD, Handley AJ, Koster RW, Castr′ en M, Smyth MA, Olasveengen T, et al. European resuscitation council guidelines for resuscitation 2015: Section 2. Adult basic life support and automated external defibrillation. Resuscitation. 2015;**95**:81-99

[22] Abella BS, Alvarado JP, Myklebust H, Edelson DP, Barry A, O'Hearn N, et al. Quality of cardiopulmonary resuscitation during in-hospital cardiac arrest. Journal of the American Medical Association. 2005;**293**(3):305-310

[23] Aufderheide TP, Lurie KG. Death by hyperventilation: A common and life-threatening problem during cardiopulmonary resuscitation. Critical Care Medicine. 2004;**32**(9): S345-S351

[24] Cheifetz IM, Craig DM, Quick G, McGovern JJ, Cannon ML, Ungerleider RM, et al. Increasing tidal volumes and pulmonary overdistention adversely affect pulmonary vascular mechanics and cardiac output in a pediatric swine model. Critical Care Medicine. 1998;**26**(4):710-716

[25] Aufderheide TP, Sigurdsson G, Pirrallo RG, Yannopoulos D, McKnite S, Von Briesen C, et al. Hyperventilation-induced hypotension during cardiopulmonary resuscitation. Circulation. 2004;**109**(16):1960-1965

[26] Gazmuri RJ, Ayoub IM, Radhakrishnan J, Motl J, Upadhyaya MP. Clinically plausible hyperventilation does not exert adverse hemodynamic effects during CPR but markedly reduces end-tidal PCO2. Resuscitation. 2012;**83**(2):259-264

[27] Risdal M, Aase SO, Stavland M, Eftestol T. Impedance-based ventilation detection during cardiopulmonary resuscitation. IEEE Transactions on Biomedical Engineering. 2007;**54**(12):2237-2245

[28] Kramer-Johansen J, Wik L, Steen PA. Advanced cardiac life support before and after tracheal intubation—direct measurements of quality. Resuscitation. 2006;**68**(1):61-69

[29] Kramer-Johansen J, Eilevstjønn J, Olasveengen TM, Tomlinson AE, Dorph E, Steen PA. Transthoracic impedance changes as a tool to detect malpositioned tracheal tubes. Resuscitation. 2008;**76**(1):11-16

[30] Edelson DP, Eilevstjønn J, Weidman EK, Retzer E, Hoek TLV, Abella BS. Capnography and chest-wall impedance algorithms for ventilation detection during cardiopulmonary resuscitation. Resuscitation. 2010;**81**(3):317-322

[31] González-Otero DM, Alonso E, Ruiz J, Aramendi E, Ruiz de Gauna S, Ayala U, et al. A simple impedance-based method for ventilation detection during cardiopulmonary resuscitation. In: Computing in Cardiology Conference (CinC); 2013. IEEE; 2013. pp. 807-810

[32] Alonso E, Ruiz J, Aramendi E, González-Otero DM, Ruiz de Gauna S, Ayala U, et al. Reliability and accuracy of the thoracic impedance signal for measuring cardiopulmonary resuscitation quality metrics. Resuscitation. 2015;**88**:28-34

[33] Edelson DP, Abella BS, Kramer-Johansen J, Wik L, Myklebust H, Barry AM, et al. Effects of compression depth and pre-shock pauses predict defibrillation failure during cardiac arrest. Resuscitation. 2006;**71**(2):137-145

[34] Gundersen K, Kvaløy JT, Kramer-Johansen J, Steen PA, Eftestøl T. Development of the probability of return of spontaneous circulation in intervals without chest compressions during out-of-hospital cardiac arrest: An observational study. BMC Medicine. 2009;**7**(1):6

[35] González-Otero DM, Ruiz de Gauna S, Ruiz J, Ayala U, Alonso E. Automatic detection of chest compression pauses using the transthoracic impedance signal. In: Computing in Cardiology (CinC). IEEE; 2012. pp. 21-24

[36] Ruiz de Gauna S, González-Otero DM, Ruiz JM, Ayala U, Alonso E, Eftestøl T, et al. Is rhythm analysis during chest compression pauses for ventilation feasible? Resuscitation. 2012;**83**:e8

[37] Ruiz J, Ayala U, Ruiz de Gauna S, Irusta U, González-Otero DM, Alonso E, et al. Feasibility of automated rhythm assessment in chest compression pauses during cardiopulmonary resuscitation. Resuscitation. 2013;**84**(9):1223-1228

[38] Idris AH, Guffey D, Pepe PE, Brown SP, Brooks SC, Callaway CW, et al. Chest compression rates and survival following out-of-hospital cardiac arrest. Critical Care Medicine. 2015;**43**(4):840-848

[39] Idris AH, Guffey D, Aufderheide TP, Brown S, Morrison LJ, Nichols P, et al. The relationship between chest compression rates and outcomes from cardiac arrest. Circulation. 2012;**125**(24):3004-3012

[40] Wik L, Kramer-Johansen J, Myklebust H, Sørebø H, Svensson L, Fellows B, et al. Quality of cardiopulmonary resuscitation during out-of-hospital cardiac arrest. Journal of the American Medical Association. 2005;**293**(3):299-304

[41] Gruber J, Stumpf D, Zapletal B, Neuhold S, Fischer H. Real-time feedback systems in CPR. Trends in Anaesthesia and Critical Care. 2012;**2**(6):287-294

[42] González-Otero DM, de Gauna SR, Ruiz JM, Gutiérrez JJ, Saiz P, Leturiondo M. Audio-visual feedback devices for chest compression quality during CPR. In: Resuscitation Aspects. Rijeka: InTech; 2017

[43] González-Otero DM. Feedback Systems for the Quality of Chest Compressions during Cardiopulmonary Resuscitation. Universidad del País Vasco (UPV/EHU); 2015

[44] Stecher FS, Olsen JA, Stickney RE, Wik L. Transthoracic impedance used to evaluate performance of cardiopulmonary resuscitation during out of hospital cardiac arrest. Resuscitation. 2008;**79**(3):432-437

[45] Aramendi E, Ayala U, Irusta U, Alonso E, Eftestøl T, Kramer-Johansen J. Suppression of the cardiopulmonary resuscitation artefacts using the instantaneous chest compression rate extracted from the thoracic impedance. Resuscitation. 2012;**83**(6):692-698

[46] Ayala U, Eftestøl T, Alonso E, Irusta U, Aramendi E, Wali S, et al. Automatic detection of chest compressions for the assessment of CPR-quality parameters. Resuscitation. 2014;**85**(7):957-963

[47] González-Otero DM, Ruiz de Gauna S, Ruiz J, Daya MR, Wik L, Russell JK, et al. Chest compression rate feedback based on transthoracic impedance. Resuscitation. 2015;**93**:82-88

[48] Brody D, Di Maio R, Crawford P, Navarro C, Anderson J. The impedance cardiogram amplitude as an indicator of cardiopulmonary resuscitation efficacy in a porcine model of cardiac arrest. Journal of the American College of Cardiology. 2011;**57**(14):E1134

[49] Di Maio R, Howe A, McCanny P, Navarro C, Crispino-O'Connell G, McIntyre A, et al. Is the impedance cardiogram a potential indicator of effective external cardiac massage in a human model? A study to establish if there is a linear correlation between the impedance cardiogram and depth in a cardiac arrest setting. Circulation. 2012; **126**(Suppl 21):A94

[50] Zhang H, Yang Z, Huang Z, Chen B, Zhang L, Li H, et al. Transthoracic impedance for the monitoring of quality of manual chest compression during cardiopulmonary resuscitation. Resuscitation. 2012;**83**(10):1281-1286

[51] Alonso E, González-Otero D, Aramendi E, de Gauna SR, Ruiz J, Ayala U, et al. Can thoracic impedance monitor the depth of chest compressions during out-of-hospital cardiopulmonary resuscitation? Resuscitation. 2014;**85**(5):637-643